VETERINARY TECHNICIANS AND ASSISTANTS

PRACTICAL CAREER GUIDES

Series Editor: Kezia Endsley

Computer Game Development & Animation, by Tracy Brown Hamilton
Craft Artists, by Marcia Santore
Culinary Arts, by Tracy Brown Hamilton
Dental Assistants and Hygienists, by Kezia Endsley
Education Professionals, by Kezia Endsley
Fine Artists, by Marcia Santore
First Responders, by Kezia Endsley
Health and Fitness Professionals, by Kezia Endsley
Information Technology (IT) Professionals, by Erik Dafforn
Medical Office Professionals, by Marcia Santore
Nursing Professionals, by Kezia Endsley
Plumbers, by Marcia Santore
Skilled Trade Professionals, by Corbin Collins
Veterinary Technicians and Assistants, by Kezia Endsley

VETERINARY TECHNICIANS AND ASSISTANTS

A Practical Career Guide

KEZIA ENDSLEY

ROWMAN & LITTLEFIELD
Lanham • Boulder • New York • London

Published by Rowman & Littlefield
An imprint of The Rowman & Littlefield Publishing Group, Inc.
4501 Forbes Boulevard, Suite 200, Lanham, Maryland 20706
www.rowman.com

6 Tinworth Street, London, SE11 5AL, United Kingdom

British Library Cataloguing in Publication Information Available

Library of Congress Cataloging-in-Publication Data

Names: Endsley, Kezia, 1968– author.
Title: Veterinary technicians and assistants : a practical career guide / Kezia Endsley.
Description: Lanham : Rowman & Littlefield Publishing Group, [2020] | Series: Practical career guides | Includes bibliographical references. | Summary: "Veterinary technicians and Assistants: A Practical Career Guide includes interviews with professionals in a field that has proven to be a stable, lucrative, and growing profession."—Provided by publisher.
Identifiers: LCCN 2019057069 (print) | LCCN 2019057070 (ebook) | ISBN 9781538133668 (paperback) | ISBN 9781538133675 (epub)
Subjects: LCSH: Animal health technicians. | Veterinary nursing—Vocational guidance. | Animal health technology—Vocational guidance.
Classification: LCC SF774.4 .E53 2020 (print) | LCC SF774.4 (ebook) | DDC 636.089/069—dc23
LC record available at https://lccn.loc.gov/2019057069
LC ebook record available at https://lccn.loc.gov/2019057070

Contents

Introduction

So You Want a Career as a Vet Technician or Assistant

*H*ave you always enjoyed connecting with and caring for animals? Well, if you think you might want to turn this passion into a career, you've come to the right book. Being a veterinary technician can be a rewarding, exciting, varied, and flexible career. Vet techs serve a critical role in helping veterinarians provide the best medical care to their animal patients. In fact, paraveterinary workers, as they are also called, are an important piece of the puzzle when it comes to providing care and comfort to animals in various settings.

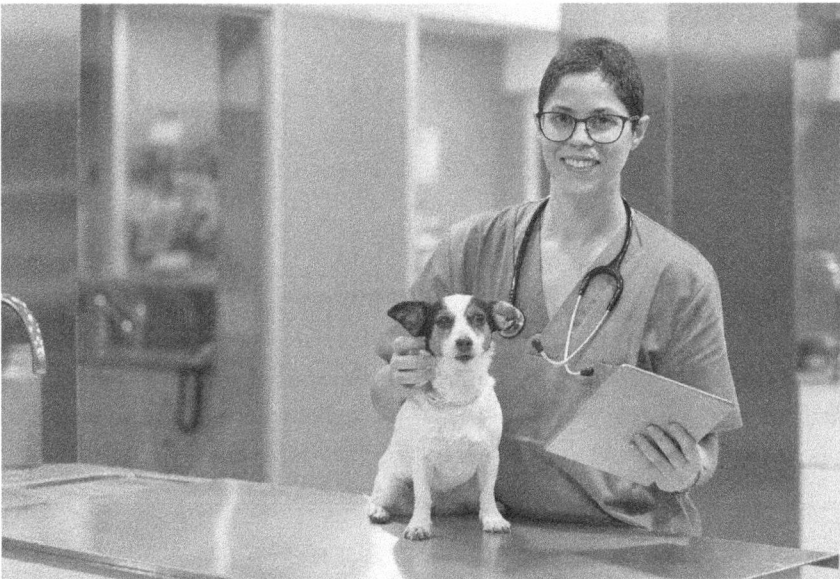

Being a vet technician is a rewarding profession when you enjoy working with animals. ©*Morsa Images/E+/Getty Images*

The day-to-day job of vet techs can vary greatly depending on the work environment in which they choose to work—from research laboratory to veterinary clinic to animal hospital and beyond (including boarding kennels, animal shelters, rescue organizations, and zoos). They work with veterinarians and other vet techs to provide medical services to animals, including such tasks as taking patient case histories from their owners, preparing animals for surgery and other care from the doctor, performing exams and prepping animals for exams, drawing blood, giving vaccinations, and much more. Chapter 1 discusses the day-to-day duties of paraveterinary workers in more detail and differentiates between the main job titles—vet technician, vet technologist, and touches on the vet assistant role.

VET TECHNICIAN VERSUS VET TECHNOLOGIST

Although this book does often use the term *vet tech* to refer to either of these variations of paraveterinary worker, there is a difference between these two careers, which will be covered in more detail later, especially in chapter 3, which discusses the educational paths.

Veterinary technicians are graduates of a two-year program accredited by the American Veterinary Medical Association (AVMA) at a community college, college, or university. They generally work in private clinical practices under the guidance of a licensed veterinarian.

Veterinary technologists are graduates of a four-year AVMA-accredited bachelor degree program. Many work in more advanced research-related jobs, usually under the guidance of a scientist and sometimes a veterinarian. They primarily work in laboratory settings.[1]

There is a lot of good news about this field, and it's a very smart career choice for anyone with a passion for animals. It's a great career for people who get energy from working with animals and aren't afraid to help scared, sick, or injured ones. Job demand is high and is expected to grow much faster than average in the United States over the next decade, as you'll learn in the next section.[2]

"My favorite part of being a vet tech is helping animals feel better. When they wake up from surgery and they are sad and scared and hurt, I can comfort them and make the pain go away and calm them. That's a great feeling!"—Sarah Jo Bouldin, RVT

The Market Today

The good news is that the US Bureau of Labor Statistics forecasts that the field of paraveterinary medicine in general will grow about 19 percent during the decade between the years 2018 and 2028, which is much faster than the average profession.[3] (See https://www.bls.gov/emp/ for a full list of employment projections.) This not only translates into job security, it also means that more new positions are being created every year.

Chapter 1 covers lots more about the job prospects of these professions, breaking down the numbers into more detail.

The Work Environment: Good, Bad, and Rewarding

In the United States, vet technicians overwhelmingly work in private clinics or animal hospitals. A smaller number work in laboratories, colleges and universities, and humane societies.[4] When they work in a laboratory or hospital setting, where care is expected to occur around the clock, they usually have a variable schedule and might be expected to work nights, weekends, and holidays. When they work for a vet clinic that is run by one or more veterinarians, the hours are more predictable, but they are often still expected to work on Saturdays.

It's important to realize at the start that paraveterinary medicine can be physically and emotionally demanding. You may witness abused animals or may need to help euthanize ("put to sleep") sick, injured, or unwanted animals. You will not be able to save every animal that comes into the clinic or hospital. If you work in a laboratory setting, you may be caring for animals that live out their lives in cages and are used for experimental purposes. Of course, if you are opposed to any of those practices, you can and should seek out like-minded organizations to work for, such as local humane societies and no-kill shelters.

Because they work with animals that are under stress and are naturally unpredictable (at least to the human mind), veterinary technologists and technicians also risk injury on the job. They can be bitten, scratched, or kicked while working with scared or aggressive animals. Injuries often happen while the technologist or technician is holding, cleaning, or restraining an animal.

You must weigh these potential negatives with the possible joy and satisfaction you'll get from treating, helping, comforting, and even saving animals as part of your daily job. When considering any career, your goal should be to find your specific nexus of interest, passion, and job demand. It is important to consider job outlook and demand, educational requirements, and other such practical matters, but remember that you'll be spending a large portion of your life in whatever career you choose, so you should also find something that you enjoy doing and are passionate about.

An important note: Regardless of the career you choose within the healthcare umbrella—as paraveterinary careers are—you need to have a lifelong curiosity and love of learning. Your education won't be over once you finish your degree or training. In fact, maintaining current certifications and meeting or exceeding continuing education requirements (usually set forth by the governing board and/or by state regulations where you practice) are very important in all the healthcare fields, including paraveterinary medicine.

What Does This Book Cover?

The book covers the pros and cons, educational requirements, projected annual wages, personality traits that match, working conditions and expectations, and more. You'll even read interviews from real professionals working in paraveterinary medicine. The goal is for you to learn enough about this profession to give you a clear view as to whether it might be a good fit for you. And if you still have questions, this book includes a number of resources where you can learn even more.

Here's a breakdown of the chapters:

- Chapter 1 explains in greater detail what vet technicians, vet technologists, and vet assistants do in their day-to-day work, the environments where you can find these people working, some pros and cons about the various career paths, the average salaries of these jobs, and the outlook in the future for these careers.
- Chapter 2 explains in detail the educational requirements, from certifications to associate's degrees to bachelor's degrees. You will learn how to go about getting experience (in the form of shadowing, internships,

and fieldwork) before you enter college as well as during your college years. You'll also learn about the certifications, licensing, and registrations required to practice safely and legally.

- Chapter 3 explains all the aspects of college and postsecondary schooling that you'll want to consider as you move forward. You will learn how to get the best education for the best deal. You will also learn a little about scholarships and financial aid and how the SAT and ACT work.
- Chapter 4 covers all aspects of the interviewing and résumé-writing processes, including writing a stellar résumé and cover letter, interviewing to your best potential, dressing for the part, communicating effectively and efficiently, and more.

Where Should You Start?

There are essentially two main levels of education and training for entry into this occupation: a four-year program for veterinary technologists and a two-year program for veterinary technicians. Typically, technologists and technicians must pass a credentialing exam and must become registered, licensed, or certified, depending on the state in which they work. This is covered in more detail in chapter 2.

As a way to get started in paraveterinary medicine, you may consider a job as a veterinary assistant, which requires only a high school diploma. Veterinary assistants perform duties such as feeding and exercising animals, bathing animals and cleaning their cages, comforting and restraining animals during procedures, and otherwise assisting veterinarians and vet technicians. Vet assistants who work in clinic settings usually make a little better than minimum wage. It's a good way to get your foot in the door and see if you really like the day-to-day work of helping animals in this manner.

Ask yourself: Are you comfortable working with large farm animals or would you rather work with house pets like cats and dogs? Are you driven to the exciting and high-pressure setting of emergency medicine or would you rather work in a more stable and predictable environment such as a standard vet clinic? Or are you interested in working with animals in a laboratory?

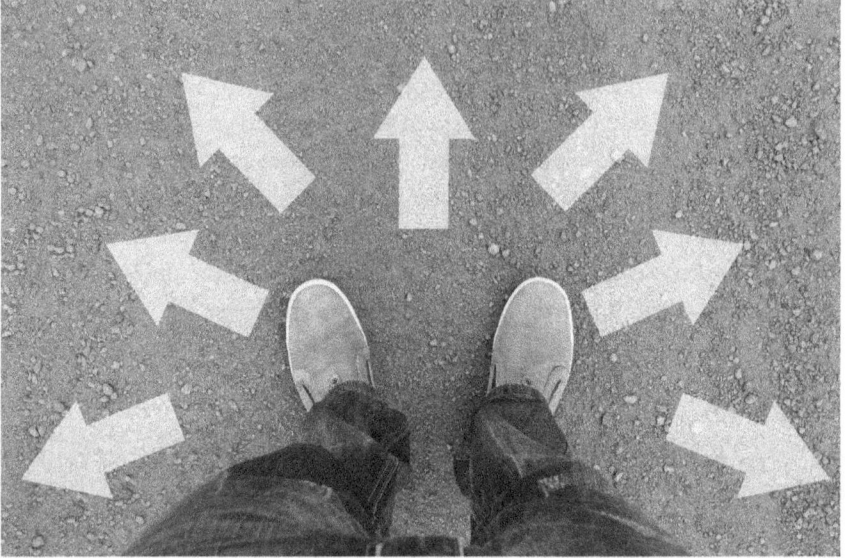

Starting your career journey can be daunting, but this book can help! ©*sergeichekman/iStock/Getty Images*

The good news is that you don't need to know the answers to these questions yet. In order to find the best fit for yourself in paraveterinary medicine, you need to understand how people in these jobs work. That's where you'll start in chapter 1.

Why Choose a Career as a Veterinary Technician or Assistant?

You learned in the introduction that paraveterinary medicine is a healthy and growing career field. You also learned a little bit about how careers in this field are split depending on your degree and level of schooling. You also were reminded that it's important to pursue a career that you enjoy, are good at, and are passionate about. You will spend a lot of your life working; it makes sense to find something you enjoy doing. Of course, you want to make money and support yourself while doing it. If you love the idea of helping animals for a living, you've come to the right book.

This chapter discusses in more detail the main responsibilities and job duties of careers in paraveterinary medicine and covers the basics of each. After reading this chapter, you should have a good understanding of these roles and can then start to determine if one of them is a good fit for you. Let's start with the veterinary assistant.

What Is a Veterinary Assistant?

The introduction mentioned that working as a veterinary assistant can be a great way to get your foot in the door and try paraveterinary medicine without committing to years of schooling. This is because the job typically requires only a high school diploma. Before committing to postsecondary schooling, you can get into a clinic, lab, or hospital setting and work with animals—and be able to determine if this is the right career path for you. Most employers also provide on-the-job training, but some will hire only those who have prior experience working with animals.[1]

MAIN RESPONSIBILITIES

Vet assistants perform everyday duties that need to be done in the clinic or lab. They assist veterinarians and veterinary technicians with routine animal care and daily tasks, including:

- Feeding and exercising the animals
- Bathing animals and cleaning their cages
- Cleaning and sterilizing equipment
- Monitoring animals and recording their findings
- Transporting animals within the facility for procedures and tests
- Comforting and restraining animals during procedures

You need to be comfortable and confident working with scared or injured animals in order to be successful as a vet assistant.

HOW HEALTHY IS THE VET ASSISTANT JOB MARKET?

The Bureau of Labor Statistics (BLS) is part of the US Department of Labor. It tracks statistical information about thousands of careers in the United States. These statistics show just how promising this career is now and in the foreseeable future:

- *Education:* High school diploma or equivalent
- *2018 median pay:* $27,540
- *Job outlook 2018–2028:* 19 percent (much faster than average)
- *Work environment:* Most work in private clinics and animal hospitals (87%); a small subset works in university research labs (5%)[2]

So the vet assistant position is a good place to start, but you may find yourself eventually wanting more responsibility, more recognition, and a higher salary. Let's move on to discussing the veterinary technician role, which is the next step on the ladder of paraveterinary medicine.

KRISTA KING

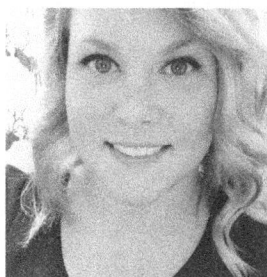

Krista King.
Courtesy of Krista King

Krista King received her associate's degree in applied science of veterinary technology in 2012. She found an entry-level job in a very small general practice, where she was able to do a large variety of jobs. She did her externship there and stayed for three or four years. Her next job was at a veterinary hospital, where the medicine and protocols were newer. She then worked in an emergency hospital, where she did three different overnight shifts for two years.

After about five years in the industry, Krista experienced burnout and hit a wall. She noticed that she wasn't seeing the joy in it anymore. She left the field for almost two years and explored other options. This time helped her focus on her career goals. She realized that veterinary medicine was what she likes to do. She came back to the animal hospital where she had previously worked and has been there about two years.

Can you explain how you became interested in being a vet tech?

I wanted to do something with animals since I was little. When I was younger, my neighbors and I used to set up a pretend vet clinic in their RV and give our stuffed animals pretend shots! After high school, I didn't really know what I wanted to do. I applied to a few colleges in my state but didn't know what to do.

I knew I wanted more hands-on with animals. I shadowed a bit before college and realized that vets don't always do the hands-on stuff like vaccines, drawing blood, and so on. The vet tech does all that. I wanted to do stuff but not have the huge responsibility of making life-and-death decisions that veterinarians have.

Can you talk about your current position? What's a typical day in your job?

I am a surgery technician. In our practice, technicians and assistants do pretty much the same things. I am not licensed at the moment, so I am technically an assistant. But I can do everything my employer allows me to do.

I get there early and set up all instruments and supplies for surgeries, calculate drugs needed, and type up surgery notes and take-home instructions. I take vitals of the patients too. When the doctor arrives, I sedate the animals. All our surgeries are in the morning. Then one surgery tech usually leaves early and one helps with afternoon appointments.

Do you think your education prepared you for your job? Do you recommend being licensed?

To a certain extent, absolutely! I tell people fresh out of school that there are a lot of things you learn in school that are actually different in practice. Animals don't always cooperate, doctors like things in different ways, etc. So you have to learn what is practical where you work.

I do recommend getting the license. I am in the process of doing that again. Mine lapsed when I was away from the field, but I want to be licensed again. I recommend doing it right after graduation, when the information is fresh in your mind. The VTNE [Veterinary Technician National Exam] test is all based on the book materials. So do it right after you graduate. There is some talk about Indiana moving to require licensing for drawing blood, vaccines, etc. Many states require this already.

What's the best part of being a vet tech?

You get to play with puppies and kittens that come in and interact with animals. You see all kinds of animals, and it's super fun. Watching them grow up and be healthy is really great.

What's the most challenging part of your job? How can people avoid burnout?

Dealing with euthanasia or sick and dying animals or emergencies are all really rough. With emergencies, you have to be very quick on your toes and try to prepare as much as you can so you can make sound life-or-death decisions. A split second can make a life-and-death difference.

How can a vet tech avoid burnout?

The best advice is to take breaks. If you feel tired or you aren't doing your best job, do take breaks. Take a vacation or take a few days. Clear your mind and don't think about work. Go somewhere that makes you happy so you can come back refreshed.

What are some things in this profession that are especially challenging right now?

The biggest thing is trying to remember everything for all the different species. You have to know what you are doing with all kinds of dogs, cats, guinea pigs, rabbits, mice, etc. Finding your confidence is a challenge too. In a practice, you are more likely to make mistakes if you don't build your confidence.

What are some characteristics of a good vet tech?

You must be personable and have good interpersonal skills. You deal with people a lot, including the time you spend educating clients. You have to be able to speak for the animals. You need a good memory. You also need to be quick and efficient.

What is the most surprising thing about your job? Is it what you expected it would be?

It is not at all what I expected! To me, it's better. You don't just hold the animals while the doctors examine them, which is what I thought originally. You do much more hands-on work with the animals—including giving shots, taking blood, cleaning teeth, giving vaccines, acting as a receptionist, talking to owners, and restraining and comforting animals.

What's next? Where do you see yourself going from here? Where do you see the field going from here?

The field is always expanding. We are always learning new things about medicines and better ways to do things. I don't expect the vet field to go anywhere. Vet medicine is here to stay. There are always new tools and such to advance the field.

My goal is to get licensed and then be the clinical trainer at my current employer as they expand. I would love to train others and help them be confident and do their jobs well.

What advice do you have for young people considering this career?

Shadow as much as you can, at different hospitals and clinics—small and large animals, with exotics, and so on—as much as you can. The practice can be very different, and you want to know if you actually like it so you don't spend all that money and waste your time. You need to see what the position is in actuality.

How can a young person prepare for a career as a vet tech while in high school?

Shadow, volunteer, and also start studying. You can find the books online and all of them are great. You can read up on the profession. This will help you in advance and give you a leg up.

What Is a Veterinary Technician?

As mentioned in the introduction, a veterinary technician is a graduate from a two-year, AVMA-accredited program at a community college, college, or university. Vet technicians work in many different settings and help the licensed

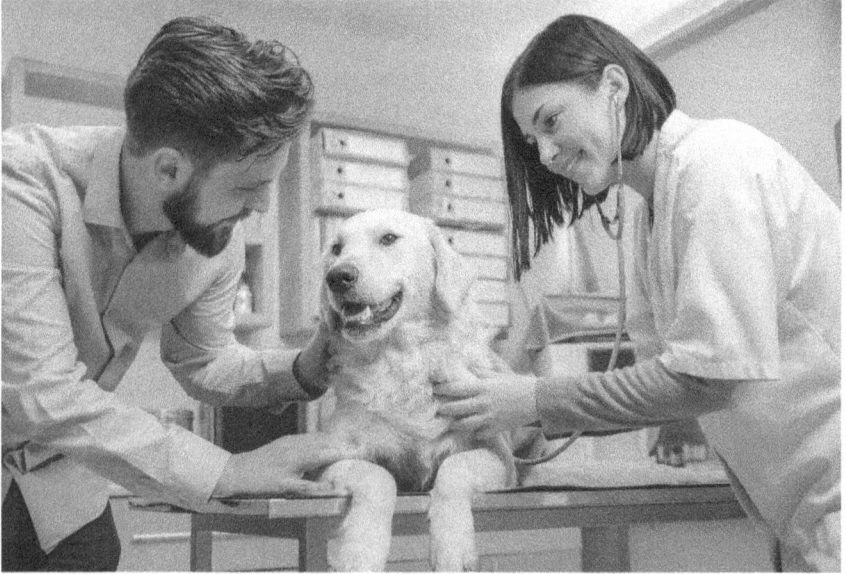

Vet technicians provide patient care to animals under the direction of a veterinarian. ©*Phoenixns/ iStock/Getty Images*

veterinarians they work with provide excellent care in the most efficient way possible. They are valuable members of the veterinary medicine team.

Depending on the type of setting they work in—a large office with many veterinarians, small office, hospital, laboratory, surgery center, rescue center, boarding kennel, zoo, and so on—their job brings special challenges and rewards. The best vet technicians have excellent communication skills and enjoy working with animals, as well as with other people.

MAIN RESPONSIBILITIES

So what do vet technicians do? Although their day-to-day work can vary greatly, some of the common tasks that vet techs may perform include:

- Observing animal conditions
- Collecting and recording patient case histories
- Collecting laboratory samples, such as blood or urine
- Performing laboratory exams
- Administering vaccines and medications, orally, anally, or via injection

- Preparing animals and instruments for surgery
- Assisting veterinarians during animal surgeries
- Bathing animals and cleaning ears, eyes, and so on
- Taking and developing X-rays
- Providing emergency care to sick or injured animals

Depending on the setting, vet technicians may also provide more extensive treatment such as dental care and special nursing care. Besides the obvious—cats and dogs—vet technicians often care for mice, birds, rats, and various types of reptiles. They may also help care for horses, cows, sheep, and other livestock if they work for a large-animal veterinarian. (There are currently eleven specialty areas of vet techs, which are discussed later in this chapter.) Vet technicians work under the supervision of a licensed veterinarian.

"I love how involved I am with patient care. I provide a ton of nursing care to these animals. I work in critical care, and I can really care for them and nurse them back to health. I do much of the hands-on tasks, rather than the vet. I am highly involved, which is very rewarding."—Courtney Waxman, RVT

In addition to good interpersonal skills, vet technicians need to have good stamina to work on their feet all day, and must be organized and reliable. The types of settings that vet technicians often work in include:

- General veterinary clinics (single-doctor and group settings)
- Specialty practices, such as exotic pet care or large-animal veterinary offices
- Settings such as zoos and large farms
- Animal hospitals
- Rescue organizations and humane societies
- Boarding kennels
- Research laboratories

Recall that to work as a vet technician, you need an associate's degree (a two-year degree) in veterinary technology. You'll usually also have to pass an exam (most likely the VTNE) and then become licensed, but the exact details depend on the state in which you work.[3] Chapters 2 and 3 cover the educational and professional certification requirements in more detail.

HOW HEALTHY IS THE VET TECHNICIAN JOB MARKET?

For anyone studying to become a vet technician, the news from the BLS is great! Employment is expected to grow 19 percent in the decade between the years 2018 and 2028, which is much faster than the average profession.[4] Vet technicians are expected to be in great demand. This increase in demand is due in part because the number of households with pets and—perhaps more importantly—*spending* on pets continues to rise. The demand will consequently increase for veterinary technologists and technicians to do laboratory work and imaging services on household pets.[5]

BLS statistics show just how promising this career is now and in the foreseeable future:

- *Education:* Usually an associate's degree, although a bachelor's degree is also common in some places; most states require vet techs to be licensed
- *2018 median pay:* $34,420
- *Job outlook 2018–2028:* 19 percent (much faster than average)
- *Work environment:* Most work in private clinics and animal hospitals (90 percent); a small subset work in university research labs (4 percent) and an even smaller number work for social advocacy organizations (2 percent)[6]

The jury is in: being a vet technician is a growing and rewarding career!

What Is a Veterinary Technologist?

As mentioned in the introduction, a veterinary technologist is a graduate from a four-year AVMA-accredited bachelor's degree program. Vet technologists can and do work in all the settings mentioned in the vet technicians section, but many work in more advanced research–related jobs, usually under the guidance of a scientist and sometimes a veterinarian. They primarily work in laboratory settings.[7]

The difference between a vet technologist and a vet technician is largely the degree. AVMA policy states that a veterinary technologist is someone with a bachelor's degree in veterinary technology.[8] However, very few states legally recognize the title veterinary technologist; in all the rest the credential granted is licensed/registered/certified veterinary technician regardless of whether the person has an associate's degree or a bachelor's degree.[9]

You can make more money with a bachelor's degree if you choose the right type of career—research, teaching, working for drug companies, working in a specialty practice, and so on. But it's just as common that you will make the same money as any other veterinary technician, at least until you prove yourself to be a more valuable asset.

MAIN RESPONSIBILITIES

In a laboratory setting, vet technologists work directly for veterinarians or scientists. They are qualified to do many tasks, including:

- Preparing testing equipment and tissue samples for examination
- Analyzing fluids and other biological materials
- Recording findings and keeping patient animal records, such as information on an animal's genealogy, weight, diet, and signs of pain
- Discussing information with veterinarians and pet owners
- Ensuring that animals are handled carefully and humanely
- Administering medications
- Doing a variety of research work

Vet technologists assist veterinarians or scientists on research projects in areas such as biomedical research, disaster preparedness, and food or product safety.

HOW HEALTHY IS THE VET TECHNOLOGIST JOB MARKET?

The BLS does not compile different statistics for vet technicians and vet technologists, but other sources state that the market is very similar to the vet technician job market, which is healthy and growing.[10]

Veterinary Technician Specialty Areas

As mentioned earlier, there are currently eleven veterinary technician specialty areas, as recognized by the National Association of Veterinary Technicians in America (NAVTA). More specialties are currently being developed, and there may be several more by the time you read this book. Check out the NAVTA website (www.navta.net) for an updated list.

To become certified as a veterinary technician specialist (VTS) in one of these areas, you first need an associate's degree in the field, significant work experience, documented continuing education, and completion of case logs and case reports. Then you will be eligible to sit for the appropriate certification exam.[11] Let's look at these specialty areas in detail.

CLINICAL PATHOLOGY VET TECHNICIAN

Clinical pathology vet technicians analyze animal bodily fluids, such as urine and blood, to identify health issues. Candidates for certification must have at least 4,000 hours (three years) of experience in the field, a yearlong case log, a skills log, five detailed case reports, and two letters of recommendation.[12]

CLINICAL PRACTICE VET TECHNICIAN

Clinical practice vet technicians provide care to animals in one of three sub-specialty areas: canine/feline, exotic companion animal, or production animal (animals raised for goods, such as food or clothing). Candidates for certification must have at least 10,000 hours (five years) of experience, fifty case logs, four case reports, and forty hours of documented continuing education.[13]

EMERGENCY AND CRITICAL CARE VET TECHNICIAN

Emergency and critical care vet technicians are trained to provide emergency care to animals that have suffered severe trauma. If you specialize in this area, you likely will work evening, overnight, and weekend shifts, since most emergency clinics operate on a twenty-four-hour basis. Candidates for certification need at least 5,760 hours (three years) of experience, a yearlong case log with at least fifty cases, four in-depth case reports, and twenty-five hours of documented continuing education.[14]

EQUINE VET TECHNICIAN

Equine vet technicians assist veterinarians who specialize in caring for horses. They are qualified to provide both routine and emergency healthcare for horses. Equine vet technicians may work in a large animal hospital or travel from farm to farm with the vet whom they assist. The American Association of Equine Veterinary Technicians oversees the certification exam.[15]

INTERNAL MEDICINE VET TECHNICIAN

Internal medicine vet technicians assist veterinarians working in a variety of subspecialties, including cardiology, neurology, and oncology. Candidates for certification must have at least 6,000 hours (three years) of experience in the field, a case log with fifty to seventy-five individual cases, four case reports, forty hours of continuing education, a completed skills checklist, and two professional letters of recommendation.[16]

VETERINARY BEHAVIOR TECHNICIAN

Veterinary behavior technicians assist in animal behavior management and modification. Candidates for certification need at least 4,000 hours (three years) of experience in the field, either a case log of fifty cases or one year of research experience, five detailed case reports, forty hours of continuing education, a completed skills checklist, and two letters of recommendation.[17]

VETERINARY SURGICAL TECHNICIAN

Veterinary surgical technicians are trained to help veterinarians with surgical procedures and to oversee preoperative and postoperative care. Candidates for certification need have at least 6,000 hours (three years) of experience in the field, with at least 4,500 hours specifically in surgical work.[18]

VET TECHNICIAN ANESTHETIST

Vet technician anesthetists are trained to help veterinary anesthesiologists and surgeons with procedures, including monitoring ventilation and sedation. Candidates for certification need 6,000 hours (three years) of experience in the field, with at least 4,500 of those hours devoted to anesthesia, a case log of fifty cases during the year of application, forty hours of continuing education in the last five calendar years, four case reports, a completed skills checklist, and two professional letters of recommendation.[19]

VETERINARY DENTAL TECHNICIAN

Veterinary dental technicians provide dental care and cleanings for animals under the supervision of a veterinarian. Candidates for certification need at least 6,000 hours of experience as a technician, with at least half those hours in dentistry, as well as fifty case logs, five detailed case reports, and forty-one hours of continuing education.[20]

VETERINARY NUTRITION TECHNICIAN

Veterinary nutrition technicians assist with the nutritional management of animals. Candidates for certification need at least 4,000 hours (three years) of experience in clinical or research-based animal nutrition, forty hours of continuing education, documented research, a yearlong case log, five detailed case reports, and two letters of recommendation.[21]

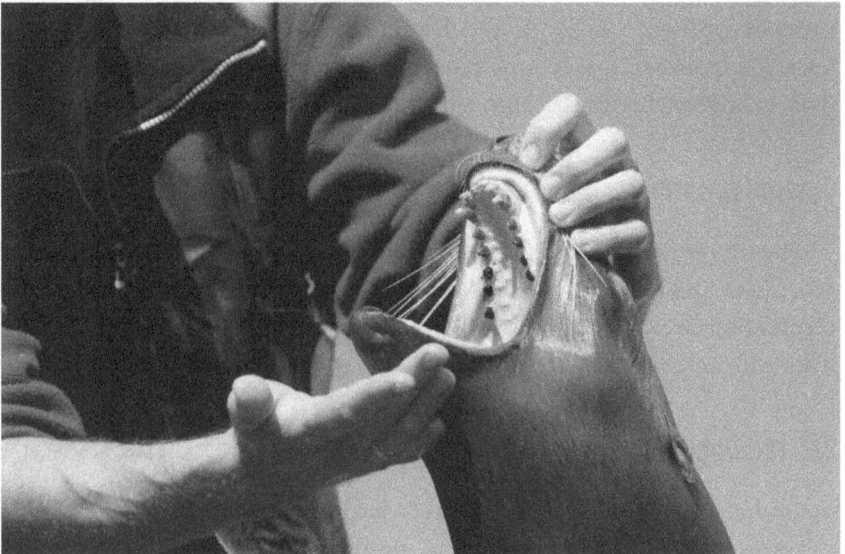

Zoo vet technicians work with exotic animal species. ©ptaxa/iStock/Getty Images

ZOO VET TECHNICIAN

Zoo vet technicians help zoo veterinarians as they work with exotic animal species. Candidates for certification need at least 10,000 hours (five years) of experience in zoological medicine, forty case log entries, forty hours of continuing education, completed skills checklists, five case reports, and two professional letters of recommendation.[22]

The Pros and Cons of Being a Vet Tech

The paraveterinary field is healthy and growing, as you've learned in this chapter. If you choose to become a vet technician or assistant, you'll likely enjoy job security. In addition to security, this is a profession that you can practice part-time without negative ramifications. Having a career in which you work with animals requires compassion and care; you will often be required to work through heart-wrenching experiences. Let's further break down some of the pros and cons.

Cons:

- *Unpredictable animals:* When an animal feels threatened or alarmed, it will try to defend itself. And when in an unfamiliar area, the situation could turn ugly, especially when the animal is sick or in pain. In these cases, animals are more likely to scratch or bite.
- *Stressful conditions:* Even though working with animals can be a great source of joy and satisfaction, dealing with them can also be a source of stress. Whether it's dealing with owners distraught over the death of their pet or witnessing animal neglect or outright abuse, you have to be ready to handle the stressful side of this profession.
- *Odd hours:* Depending on the setting in which they work, vet technicians may be expected to work on nights and/or weekends. Vet hospitals typically have vet technicians on hand caring for animals twenty-four hours a day.
- *Pay:* The degree and credentials can be expensive to obtain compared to how much you can make as a vet tech. This debt-to-income ratio is particularly high in veterinary medicine. That's true for technicians, technologists, and veterinarians.

- *Physically taxing:* You will be on your feet and working hands-on with animals all day. This can lead to chronic physical issues, such as back pain, that you need to be ready to manage and treat.

Pros:

- *Meaningful rewards:* This is the number-one reason people in veterinary medicine are drawn to the profession! Nothing can describe the feeling of helping an animal in pain, comforting an animal who is frightened, sending a once very sick animal home wagging its tail, or helping owners better understand and care for their pets. The emotional rewards are real, frequent, and meaningful.
- *Flexibility:* Vet technicians have the flexibility to work in a diverse set of environments, not just in the local veterinarian's office. This position is perfect for those who desire a continuously changing environment. You can work different shifts and different positions, depending on the hours you need, and this can change over your career as your needs change.
- *Exciting work environment:* As a vet technician, your work environment changes every day. It's not a mundane office job. Interaction with various animals and the completion of numerous tasks throughout the day ensures an extremely productive and rewarding workday.
- *Hands-on work:* As a vet technician, you will be directly involved with patient care, providing lots of hands-on nursing care to the animals you serve.
- *Job growth and security:* Vet technicians are in high demand and the field continues to grow.

Some of these cons can be avoided depending on the setting in which you choose to work. If odd hours are a concern for you, for example, you can work in a private vet office without a hospital. Other cons, such as dealing emotionally with dying or neglected animals, are difficult or impossible to avoid. The best way to know if you can handle any stressful situation is to put yourself there. Volunteer at a local animal shelter, hospital, or clinic and spend time seeing what the vet techs really do, day in and day out.

DANIELLE FULLER

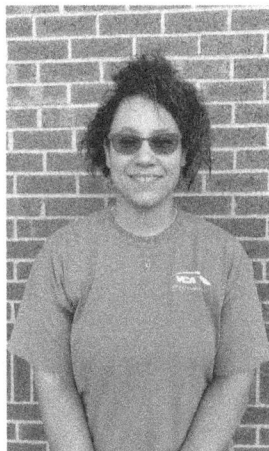

Danielle Fuller.
Courtesy of Danielle Fuller

About thirteen years ago, Danielle Fuller was just out of college, working with horses as a barn manager. She had ridden horses for the cavalry and was in the ROTC during college. Her degree was a bachelor of history/sociology, and she wasn't sure what she wanted to do until she realized she could do medicine with horses! She worked with horses as a vet assistant for two years while pursuing her vet technology degree.

Because her husband traveled a lot, she moved from large animal to small animal practices while she was in veterinary technology school and continued to work in the Washington, DC, area as an assistant vet technician in a clinic setting. She got her degree in 2010 and then moved to Indiana. She started working at a local private veterinary office, where she still works part-time. In July 2019, she also took a job at VCA Advanced Veterinary Care Center, where she is an anesthesiologist for MRI and CT.

Can you talk about your current position?

In the standard clinic setting, I really enjoy assisting with surgeries. I especially enjoy dentistry, so I was able to do pretty much all the dental cleanings. I also assisted in lots of different surgeries, such as mass removals, spays, neuters, and emergency surgeries.

We don't cover wellness at VCA, which is more like an animal hospital. I work mainly as the anesthesiologist for MRI, CT, and ultrasound. My job is called a versa-tech, because I can jump into different departments as needed. I can rotate through the ICW (intensive care ward), oncology department, and so on. I place IV catheters, help with fluids, provide patient care, etc.

This is different medicine than I have been doing, because now I'm dealing with older and sicker patients. I like seeing so many aspects of vet medicine and am now learning new things. It's a lot of learning, which I enjoy!

Do you think education prepared you for your job?

Yes, I do. They have a couple of different options—online program or veterinary/school setting. I did a little bit of both. There is lots of continuing education too. Conferences and such, as well as online.

Most schools require you to work at or volunteer at a clinic before you get your degree, which is very helpful. I felt prepared because of this, with perhaps the exception of exotic animals. I did not get a lot of exotic and zoo medicine. You get a rotation of this, but it's not enough—but they do have a specialty in it. I've also been considering getting a specialty in vet technology for anesthesiology.

What's the best part of being a vet technician?

Taking care of animals. Making a difference in the pet's life and a family's life. With wellness especially, you are helping them have a healthy family member.

It's also a good, flexible profession for people with families. You can work different shifts and different positions, depending on the hours you need, and that can change over your career as your needs change too.

What are some issues in this profession that are especially challenging?

The biggest challenges for me are client expectations. Some get upset if the outcome isn't what they hoped for. Some animals come in very sick, and there are lots of emotions that happen. Euthanasia is difficult too.

What are some characteristics of a good vet technician?

People skills are important. You must be calm and handle pressure well. Steady hands are important too! Multitasking is important. Vet techs help with physical therapy, dentistry, radiography, anesthesia, nursing care, etc., which you wouldn't do really on the human side all at once. You have to learn all that. You're only as good as your weakest link.

What advice do you have for young people considering this career?

You should know that there are lots of aspects to veterinary medicine. Try to see as much of it as possible before you pick which path to go into. There is so much out there and many different paths, so look into the one that interests you the most.

How can a young person prepare for a career as a vet technician while in high school?

Many clinics allow kids to come in and job shadow. You can come in, tour, and see how it works. Volunteer where you can, such as at a shelter. They have age restrictions, but it usually is an option for high schoolers. Volunteer at a clinic too—help clean up and see how it works there. Make sure you ask questions.

Any last thoughts?

Knowing how many possibilities there are in the veterinary medicine field is really helpful. Be sure to continue to learn—don't settle!

Am I Right for This Profession?

Ask yourself these questions:

- Do I like meeting, talking with, working with, and helping people? (Even though you work with animals, a large part of your job will be patient education and communicating with and working with the team of vets and vet techs.)
- Am I detail oriented and able to handle multiple tasks at once?
- Am I a critical thinker, and can I act quickly on my feet?
- Am I ready to spend most of my working day on my feet?
- Do I enjoy learning about biology, anatomy, and science in general? Am I a lifelong learner?
- Can I handle the emotional issues that accompany dealing with sick animals and owners who might not be able to give them the care they need?
- Am I ready to give advice that might not be followed even if it's best for my patients? Can I accept that not everyone will do what's best for their animals?

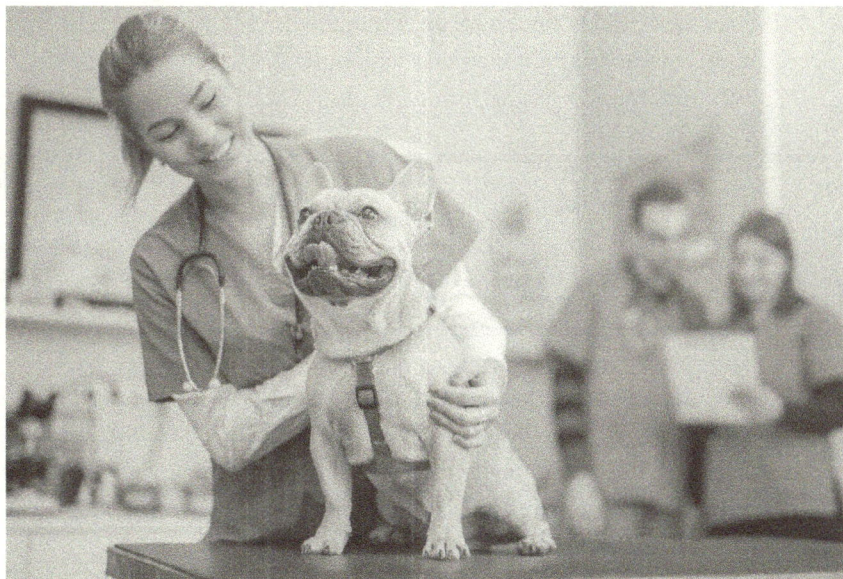

Veterinary medicine involves collaborative and cooperative work with the whole team. ©DjelicS/E+/ Getty Images

- Am I comfortable around animals who are sick or disabled? Am I able to handle being present when animals pass away?

If the answer to any of these questions is an adamant *no*, you might want to consider a different path. However, keep in mind that many of these skills can be learned and honed if you have the right attitude and a passion for the field.

Characteristics of a Great Vet Technician

Regardless of the source you turn to, you'll find the same basic characteristics used to describe a great vet technician. They all boil down to these:

- Have a compassionate, empathetic nature
- Be a good communicator and have good interpersonal skills
- Be detail oriented and organized
- Be adaptable
- Be emotionally stable and calm
- Have physical and mental endurance
- Be a quick thinker (and have great judgment)
- Be eager to learn and not afraid to ask questions
- Feel comfortable working with all kinds of animals

"Make sure you're not going into this field for the money, because it doesn't pay what human medicine does. We do it because it's a calling, not because it's going to make us the big bucks."—Erin Lee Arvin, RVT

If you pursue a career that fundamentally conflicts with the person you are, you won't be good at it and you won't be happy. Don't make that mistake. If you need help in determining your key personality factors, you can take a career counseling questionnaire to find out more. You can find many online or ask your school guidance counselor for reputable sources.

Summary

In this chapter, you learned a lot about the different roles that veterinary technicians can take, including the specialties you can focus on. You've learned about what vet technicians and assistants in these roles do in their day-to-day work, the environments where you can find these people working, some pros and cons about each career path, the average salaries of these jobs, and the outlook in the future for these careers. You hopefully even contemplated some questions about whether your personal likes and preferences meld well with these jobs. At this time, you should have a good idea what this career looks like. Are you starting to get excited about being a vet technician or assistant? If not, that's okay, as there's still time.

An important takeaway from this chapter is that no matter which area of paraveterinary medicine you decide to pursue, keep in mind that maintaining licensure and meeting continuing education requirements is very important. Advances in understanding in the fields of medicine, pharmacology, nutrition, and more are continuous, and it's vitally important that you keep apprised of what's happening in your field. You need to have a lifelong love of learning to succeed in this field.

Chapter 2 dives into forming a plan for your future, covering everything there is to know about educational requirements, certifications, internship and clinical requirements, and more. You'll learn about finding summer jobs and making the most of volunteer work as well. The goal is for you to set yourself apart—and above—the rest.

2

Forming a Career Plan

Now that you have some idea about what vet technicians do and the types of environment they work in—or maybe you even know that you want to start pursing a career in this field—it's time to formulate a career plan. For you organized folks out there, this can be a helpful and energizing process. If you're not a naturally organized person, or if the idea of looking ahead and building a plan to adulthood scares you, you are not alone. That's what this chapter is for.

After discussing ways to develop a career plan—there is more than one way to do this!—the chapter dives into the various educational requirements of this profession. Finally, it looks at how you can gain experience through internships, volunteering, clinic work, shadowing, and more. Yes, experience will look good on your résumé, and in some cases it's even required, but even more important, getting out there and experiencing a job in various settings is the best way to determine whether it's really something that you will enjoy. When you find a career that you truly enjoy, it will rarely feel like work at all.

If you still aren't sure if a career in paraveterinary medicine is right for you, try a self-assessment questionnaire or a career aptitude test. There are many good ones on the web. As an example, the career resource website Monster.com includes free self-assessment tools at www.monster.com/career-advice/article /best-free-career-assessment-tools. The Princeton Review also has a very good aptitude test geared toward high schoolers at https://www.princetonreview .com/quiz/career-quiz.

Your ultimate goal should be to match your personal interests and goals with your preparation plan for college and career. Practice articulating your plans and goals to others. When you feel comfortable doing this, you likely have a good grasp of your goals and your plan to reach them.

Planning the Plan

You are on a fact-finding mission of sorts. A career fact-finding plan, no matter what the field, should include these main steps:

- Take some time to consider and jot down your interests and personality traits. Are you a people person, or do you get energy from being alone? Are you creative or analytical? Are you outgoing or shy? Are you organized or creative—or a little of both? Take a career counseling questionnaire (found online or in your guidance counselor's office) to find out more. Consider whether your personal likes and preferences meld well with the jobs you are considering.
- Find out as much as you can about the day-to-day of the job. In what kinds of environments is it performed? Whom will you work with? How demanding is the job? What are the challenges? Chapter 1 of this book is designed to help you in this regard.
- Find out about educational requirements and schooling expectations. Will you be able to meet any rigorous requirements? This chapter and the next will help you understand the educational paths and licensing requirements.
- Seek out opportunities to volunteer or shadow professionals doing the job. Use your critical thinking skills to ask questions and consider whether this is the right environment for you. This chapter also discusses ways to find internships, summer jobs, and other job-related experiences.
- Look into student aid, grants, scholarships, and other ways you can get help to pay for schooling. It's not just about student aid and scholarships, either. Some larger organizations will pay employees to go back to school to get further degrees.
- Build a timetable for taking required exams such as the SAT and ACT, applying to schools, visiting schools, and making your decision. You should write down all the important deadlines and have them at the ready when you need them.
- Continue to look for employment that matters during your college years—internships and work experiences that help you get hands-on experience in and knowledge about your intended career.
- Find a mentor who is currently practicing in your field of interest. This person can be a great source of information, education, and connec-

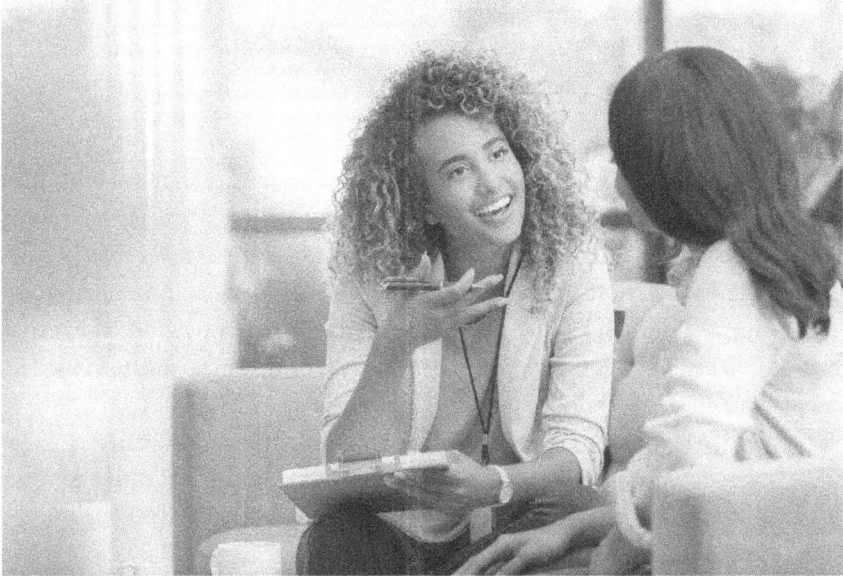

A mentor can help you figure out which way to go with your career aspirations. ©SDI Productions/ E+/Getty Images

tions. Don't expect a job (at least not at first); just build a relationship with someone who wants to pass along his or her wisdom and experience. Coffee meetings or even e-mails are a great way to start.

> "There are lots of aspects to veterinary medicine. Try to see as much of it as possible before you pick which path to go into. There is so much out there and many different paths, so look into the areas that interest you the most."—Danielle Fuller

Where to Go for Help

If you aren't sure where to start, your local library, school library, and guidance counselor's office are great places to begin. Search your local or school library for resources about finding a career path and finding the right schooling that fits your needs and budget. Make an appointment with or email a counselor to ask about taking career interest questionnaires. With a little prodding, you'll be directed to lots of good information online and elsewhere. You can start your research with these four sites:

- The Bureau of Labor Statistics' Career Outlook site at www.bls.gov/careeroutlook/home.htm doesn't just track job statistics, as you learned in chapter 1. An entire section of the BLS website is dedicated to helping young adults looking to uncover their interests and to match those interests with jobs currently in the market. Check out the section called "Career Planning for High Schoolers." Information is updated based on career trends and jobs in demand as well.
- The Mapping Your Future site at www.mappingyourfuture.org helps you determine a career path and then helps you map out a plan to reach those goals. It includes tips on preparing for college, paying for college, job hunting, résumé writing, and more.
- The Education Planner site at www.educationplanner.org has separate sections for students, parents, and counselors. It breaks down the task of planning your career goals into simple, easy-to-understand steps. You can find personality assessments, get tips on preparing for school, learn from some Q&As from counselors, download and use a planner worksheet, read about how to finance your education, and more.
- The TeenLife site at www.teenlife.com calls itself "the leading source for college preparation" and includes lots of information about summer programs, gap year programs, community service, and more. Promoting the belief that spending time out "in the world" outside of the classroom can help students do better in school, find a better fit in terms of career, and even interview better with colleges, this site contains lots of links to volunteer and summer programs.

Use these sites as jumping-off points and don't be afraid to reach out to a real person, such as a guidance counselor, if you're feeling overwhelmed.

KATIE STALDER

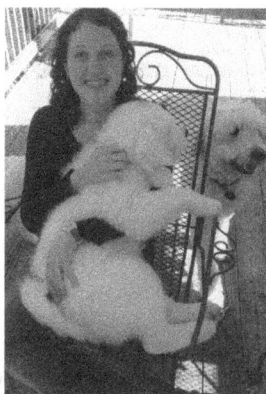

Katie Stalder.
Courtesy of Katie Stalder

Katie Stalder graduated with her veterinary technology degree in 2011. She then passed the national and state tests and became registered. She has worked in the industry consistently except during the one and a half years she took off when she had a baby.

Her residence of Asheville, North Carolina, was flooded with vet technicians, so it was hard to find a full-time position at first. She worked part-time at several different places, including at a rescue shelter as the cat intake coordinator. She also worked part-time at an animal hospital with exotics. She also worked part-time at an ER clinic for about four years and a pathology lab part-time.

When she went full-time, it was in the ER in after-hours care. She worked there for three years and then moved into specialty care in cardiology. That work consumed about sixty to seventy hours a week.

Since 2017 Katie has been working at a day practice that cares for cats and dogs. This more predictable schedule works better for her with her child and her family.

Can you explain how you became interested in becoming a vet technician?

I was working at a grooming and day care facility in Asheville with a person who was in the tech program. I was a little older. I had graduated high school in 2001 and this was 2008. I didn't think I was smart enough, but with her encouragement, I applied to vet school and I was able to go right into school without taking the prerequisites. That person worked with large animals, which was cool and interesting to me, to expand my focus.

What's a typical day in your job?

At the clinic, I get in at 8:00 a.m. I am surgery tech, so I get the pre-op blood work on the patients having surgery, calculate their meds, work with other techs who might not be registered, so I guide them. When the surgeries are complete, I do aftercare with the animals, note taking, and billing. During the surgeries, I administer meds, place an IV catheter, induce, intubate, anesthesia, shaving, clean teeth, monitor anesthesia and recovery. A huge part of my job is training new hires. Only the registered techs can administer anesthesia and monitor it.

Do you think education prepared you for your job? Do you recommend licensing?

The education was intense and profound. It's two solid years intensive preparation. It's essential. I did my second-year clinical practice within the local humane society. We were able to practice on shelter animals and learn a lot. I gained a real medical understanding and a frame of reference. Some people work in hospitals first and then go to school, but I did the opposite, so school was especially challenging.

What are the more challenging parts of being a vet technician?

You don't get paid enough for what you do, that's for sure. Not as much as a nurse. And nurses can focus on one or a few things. Vet techs are nurses who work with animals and our skills are widely varied. We have to know about radiology, anesthesia, emergency care, pathology, urinalysis, hematology analysis, etc. You have to know a lot, and about different types of animals too.

Also, it's hard on the body. You must be strong and flexible to be able to handle and restrain animals. You are on your feet all day also. Neck and back pain and carpal tunnel are common. Stay fit and strong. I don't see a lot of people over forty in this job. As vet techs age, they go into management, hiring, training, etc.

What's the best part of being a vet technician?

When I am holding an animal and helping them and comforting them! Being paid for helping animals is wonderful. Being able to speak to animals and help them through a stressful ordeal is great.

How can people avoid burnout in this job?

Self-care is so important. This job is hard on your emotions. Emergency especially, working twenty-hour shifts, can be so physically and mentally taxing.

Good employers will not work their techs to death. Find a good employer who treats their staff well. They have to care about their employees' well-being and equip their employees to deal with the stresses of the job. Compassion fatigue is a big deal, for example, and education can help.

What are some things in this profession that are especially challenging right now?

The degree is expensive to get, yet we don't make very much money. The same is true with vets (doctors). It costs a lot to get the degree and you can have a lot of debt. There is not as much respect for people who work in vet medicine.

I wish that the field supported the specialty licensing for vet techs better. There are sixteen or so specialty areas, including internal med, behavior, equine, exotic, etc. It's very hard and expensive to get licensing, and they don't make much more money. I wish it was more reasonable to accomplish and was actually financially worth it. The incentive to do it needs to be greater. You can get extra money lecturing, but it's not great. We don't want the best people to leave the field.

What are some characteristics of a good vet technician?

You must have strength, good flexibility, and coordination. Also a strong emotional self-awareness to know when you need help. Compassion is important, but it can hurt you in the long run. You have to be able to deal with the tragic events that happen. You have to be able to cope with the tragedies or you won't last very long.

What is the most surprising thing about your job? Is it what you expected it would be?

The surprising thing is that it's really about the people too. You work on a team and must get along with them. People who want to work with animals don't always want to work with people. You have to develop your interpersonal skills. Human interaction is important in this job. You have to learn to work with other people. Good interpersonal skills are important for client education.

Where do you see yourself going from here? Where do you see the field going from here?

The field is changing toward requiring more education, but I don't know how far that will go. The more highly educated vet techs are, the more they have to be paid, which means vets have to charge more, etc. There is only so much people are willing to pay for their pets, and pet insurance is not a big thing yet. It's a slow process.

As far as my future, I want to do pet boarding as my own business, or be in leadership.

What advice do you have for young people considering this career?

Get a doctorate if you can. Half of my paycheck goes to childcare. If you want a family, get a doctorate.

How can a young person prepare for a career as a vet technician while in high school?

Volunteer at rescue shelters or humane societies. Learn the animal language and physical cues; that will really help you. You need to get over fear of being bitten and scratched and deal with the sadness. My years in rescue really helped me and taught me very quickly how to handle animals. It's important to be able to speak the animals' language. You learn how to handle, feed, etc. You learn very fast.

You'll learn if you can actually handle it as well.

Making High School Count

If you are interested in working in some capacity in veterinary medicine, there are some basic yet important things you can do while in high school to position yourself in the most advantageous way. Remember—it's not just about having the best application; it's also about figuring out what professions you actually would enjoy doing and which ones don't suit you.

- Load up on the sciences, especially biology and anatomy. A head start in anatomy, biology, and/or physiology will be a big help.
- Be comfortable using all kinds of computer software.
- Learn first aid and CPR. You'll need these important skills regardless of your profession.
- Hone your communication skills in English, speech, and debate. You'll need them to speak with everyone from veterinarians to animal owners to coworkers.
- Volunteer in as many settings as you can. Read on to learn more about this important aspect of career planning.

Educational Requirements

There are two main levels of veterinary services education that you can obtain after earning your high school diploma: a four-year bachelor's degree program in veterinary technology for veterinary technologists or a two-year associate's degree program in veterinary technology for veterinary technicians. After finishing their schooling, technologists and technicians alike usually have to pass an exam (most likely the Veterinary Technician National Exam) and then must become registered, licensed, or certified, but this does depend on the state in which they work.[1] Let's start by discussing the process of finding a good vet technology program.

FINDING AN ACCREDITED SCHOOL

Regardless of whether you pursue the associate's degree or the bachelor's degree, it's important that the school or college you attend be recognized and accredited by the American Veterinary Medical Association, which is the organization that provides educational accreditation and certification programs in the veterinary field with the goal to "protect and elevate the quality of veterinary care."[2] If you obtain your schooling from a program that is not accredited by the AVMA, you cannot sit for the credentialing exams in most states.

Keep in mind that community colleges and technical schools can be a much cheaper way (as much as half the cost) to earn the same degree, and as long as those programs are accredited by the AVMA, it won't matter to potential employers that you didn't attend a more well-known university.

In 2019 there were more than two hundred veterinary technology programs in the United States and Canada that were accredited by the AVMA. Most of these programs offered a two-year associate's degree for veterinary technicians, and about twenty of them offered a four-year bachelor's degree in veterinary technology.[3] Ten of the schools offered coursework through distance learning.[4] Some of the typical classes you would take include the following:

- Basic Biology
- Introduction to Veterinary Technology
- Small Animal Husbandry and Restraint
- Veterinary Anatomy and Physiology
- Large Animal Nursing and Medicine
- Laboratory and Exotic Animal Care and Nursing
- Veterinary Anesthesia and Surgical Nursing
- Animal Diseases

Remember, if you are interested in becoming a veterinary technologist or technician and are still in middle or high school, you should take classes in biology and other sciences, as well as math.

Visit the AVMA website at www.avma.org/ProfessionalDevelopment/Education /Accreditation/Programs/Pages/vettech-programs.aspx for an updated and complete list of vet tech programs that have been accredited by the Committee on Veterinary Technician Education and Activities (CVTEA), which is the accrediting arm of the AVMA. The site provides links to each state so you can see the accredited programs in your area. This is a good place to start to find a school that's accredited *and* meets your educational and financial needs.

LICENSES AND CERTIFICATIONS

Although each state regulates veterinary technologists and technicians differently, most candidates must pass a credentialing exam to be recognized as vet techs by their state. Most states require vet technicians to pass the VTNE, a computer-based exam that is given three times a year at testing centers throughout the United States and Canada.

An important clarification: There is no national licensing exam. Passing the VTNE does not in and of itself grant certification. This test is simply the most widely used and well-known method that many states and professional associations use as proof of knowledge. Actual credentials are given by state governmental agencies or professional associations.[5] Credentials granted by state agencies are valid only in the state in which they were granted.

Even though it is not legally required in every state, passing the VTNE shows potential employers that you are capable of performing the duties required. Many places of employment (and certain states) might require this in order to be considered for a job. See https://cdn.ymaws.com/www.navta.net/resource/resmgr/vn_initiative /VeterinaryNursingMap.html for a clickable map of the United States that links to each state's certification requirements.

For vet technologists and technicians who want to work in a research facility, the American Association for Laboratory Animal Science (AALAS)— see http://www.aalas.org—offers three levels of certification: assistant laboratory animal technician, laboratory animal technician, and laboratory animal technologist.

WHAT'S THE DIFFERENCE BETWEEN
ACCREDITATION AND CERTIFICATION?

The terms *accreditation* and *certification* can be confusing, and people often mix them up and use them incorrectly, contributing to the overall confusion. Accreditation is the act of officially recognizing an organizational body, person, or educational facility as having a particular status or being qualified to perform a particular activity; for example, schools and colleges are accredited.

Certification, on the other hand, is the process of confirming that a person has certain skills or knowledge. This is usually provided by some third-party review, assessment, or educational body. (In the case of vet techs, this is usually handled by state governmental agencies.) Individuals, not organizations, are certified. This also might be referred to as being licensed.

Duties and responsibilities of vet techs vary by state, but they must demonstrate to prospective employers that they are competent in animal husbandry, health and welfare, and management. For a comprehensive list of allowable duties and credential requirements per state, visit www.avma.org/Advocacy /StateAndLocal/Pages/scope-vet-assistant-duties.aspx.

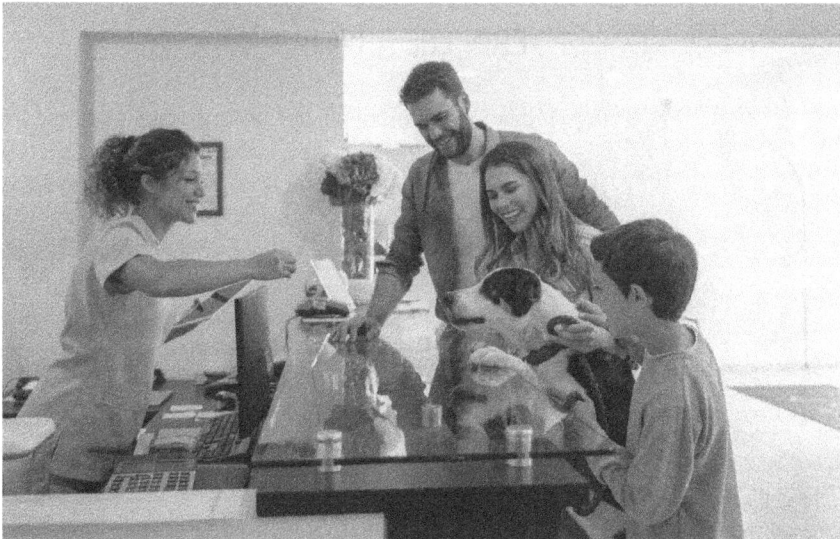

Getting certified and licensed as a vet technician takes commitment, hard work, and devotion.
©andresr/E+/Getty Images

VET TECHNICIAN VERSUS VET TECHNOLOGIST: PROS AND CONS

The decision to pursue the associate's degree or the bachelor's degree is a personal choice that is affected by many financial and personal issues (time and money, essentially). Both degrees will prepare you to take the VTNE exam, and they are similar in others ways as well.

The duties of a veterinary technologist, who goes to school two additional years, are often very close to the same as the veterinary technician who has a two-year degree. These duties include surgical assistance, medications, lab work, paperwork, and even customer education. In addition, the median salary for the vet technologist position is very close to the vet technician (around $32,500 and opposed to $32,000).[6] So one could make a salient argument that the payoff of the additional two years of schooling is negligible.

Exceptions to this may be if you plan on eventually attending veterinary school to get your DVM or if your state or area does reward the veterinary technologist degree with higher pay. In these cases, it may be better to pursue the four-year degree.

ERIN LEE ARVIN

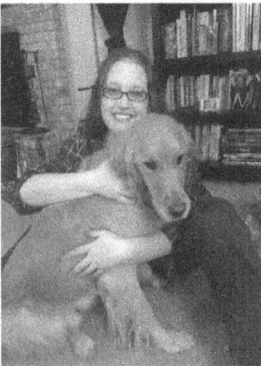

Erin Lee Arvin.
Courtesy of Erin Lee Arvin

Erin Lee Arvin got her first BA in women's studies with a minor in English from a liberal arts college. She took a job in a small mom-and-pop pet shop and realized that she liked creepy crawlies, exotics, and customer education. Someone suggested she go to vet tech school, so she got her associate's in applied science in veterinary technology. She passed the VTNE test and became licensed in 2012. The clinic where she did her externship was a mixed-animal practice, but didn't have a spot for a full-time registered veterinary technician (RVT), so she worked half as a receptionist and half as an RVT. Eventually, she was asked to specialize in practice management, and seven years later she is still enjoying that role. She maintains her RVT license but primarily deals in the administration role. She is also on the advisory board for the Central Nine Career Center Veterinary Careers, and lectures there and at the Humane Society. She also participates in other community outreach programs designed to bring middle school, high school, and college-aged students into the field.

Can you explain how you became interested in becoming a vet technician?

I became interested in veterinary medicine when I worked with a senior citizen at the pet shop who "did vet teching" back in the 1970s, when Indiana didn't require schooling or passing boards to call yourself a vet tech. She said, "Hey, I think you'd be good at this." After seeing a lot of animals surrendered to our pet shop for husbandry issues that could've been easily corrected with proper education, I realized how important vet med is, no matter how big (or small) the pet, from Dubia cockroaches to alligators.

What is a typical day in your job?

A typical day for me includes liaising with students and externs to make sure they are hitting their vet assistant or vet tech competencies for their classes; liaising with instructors at vet tech and high schools to provide feedback on their students placed with us; submitting payroll; arbitration for client or staff issues and ensuring issues are resolved in a timely and appropriate manner; getting inevitably pulled into rooms for pinch-hitting RVT skills (venipuncture, filling scripts, client education, euthanasia, etc.); dealing with vendors and merchants; accounts receivable; managing the large animal billing and client base; acting as a go-between with the many rescues, animal control organizations, wildlife rehabilitators, and shelters; working with pet insurance companies to get client claims submitted and paid; creating handouts and client education materials to disseminate information; ensuring the clinic is adhering to fear-free medicine; and promoting the human-animal bond.

What is the best part of your job?

The best part of my job is my work with students. I love being able to see the passion that young people have when they are on fire for veterinary medicine and can't wait to start their careers! These young men and women are the future of my field, so I want to make sure not only do they have a reasonable expectation of what they're getting themselves into, but also that the best and brightest end up in veterinary medicine and we don't lose them to human medicine.

What is the most challenging part of your job?

The most challenging part of my job is our work with animal control and rescue organizations. The people themselves are fabulous, passionate, yet entirely overwhelmed.

Animal controls in particular get painted with the brush that they are government pawns who don't care, but nothing could be further from the truth. They deal with horrible, soul-sucking cases and still somehow keep plugging away at the work, day after day. Seeing cases of starvation, senseless pet deaths, both active and passive neglect, and abuse can take a toll on you for sure.

What is the most surprising thing about this profession that you've seen?

The most surprising thing about veterinary medicine is just how much you can do in the field—I had no idea what I could do with even a vet tech degree, let alone what DVMs can do. You can work in private practice (be it small animal, mixed-animal, or large animal); academia; 4-H; work in a specialty practice with dermatology, ultrasound, emergency—you name it! You can work with wildlife rehabilitators; zoos; private collectors or aquariums; shelters or rescues; in research; for large-scale breeding operations such as hog or cattle farms; private training; horse racing; federal government work for the military, FDA, or USDA— the possibilities are endless!

Did your education prepare you for the job?

That's a loaded question. In some ways my education prepared me for the job; in other ways not. I will say my education prepared me for what my head would need, but not my heart. I got the basic knowledge about pharmacology, surgical and medical nursing, and what to do and what not to do. What it didn't prepare me for are the emotional expenditures that vet med requires, and how hard it is to maintain a work-life balance, fight compassion fatigue, and keep loving the human race when you see what they are capable of in regard to their furry and feathered friends.

Is the job what you expected?

Absolutely not. I was so green when I started in this field that even with shadowing at a clinic in Carmel during tech school, I didn't get an accurate representation of how bonkers veterinary medicine is. People expect crazy and ridiculous things of vet med and its staff that they never expect from our human compatriots. No one asks a human doctor to drop off a prescription at their home because the client's kid has a soccer game. No one asks the human pharmacy to "stay open later" or asks their dentist if they can throw in extractions for free. People never bring their dog to a human doctor and then ask them to see if something "looks infected." People don't want to respect the breadth of veterinarians' knowledge and realize that in addition to as much schooling and debt as human docs go through, vets know not just one species, but sometimes dozens. That's a lot of TPRs (temperature, pulse, and respiration) to memorize!

Where do you see yourself going from here? Where do you see the field going from here?

I am working toward my CVPM, a certified veterinary practice manager. I have about a year's worth more of work before I will be ready to send in the massive and daunting application and sit for the examination. I think the future of veterinary medicine is very uncertain. As people are focusing more on technology and less on brick-and-mortar, people are going to start looking toward telemedicine and online sources for products, from food to supplements and scripts. I believe this shift hurts the client-patient relationship and devalues the work vets and their teams provide. Also, I believe that veterinary medicine will move forward in the fields of pain management and behavior, and practices such as ear cropping, tail docking, and declaws will fall out of popularity. Hopefully, the trend toward spay/neuter and strong TNR (trap, neuter, return) programs will continue.

What is your advice for a young person considering this career?

For a young person considering this field, I would tell them to get into different environments as early and as often as possible. Walk dogs at the local humane society to see how they operate. See if you can volunteer at your local vet to help out during the summers. Learn the sights and smells and terms of a vet clinic or kennel or barn. And for certain make sure you're not going into this field for the money, because it doesn't pay what human medicine does. We do it because it's a calling, not because it's going to make us the big bucks.

EXPERIENCE-RELATED REQUIREMENTS

It's important to realize that any healthcare-related education you pursue will require hours of clinical work, which—in the case of veterinary medicine— includes hands-on practice with animal patients in real-world settings. The number of hours of clinical experience you need depends on the degree you pursue, as well as your own state's requirements. You might wonder how you can prepare for that experience and use fieldwork and/or internships to test the waters so you can determine whether veterinary medicine really is for you.

This section helps point you to ways in which you can gain critical experience in the veterinary field before and during the time you're pursuing your education. This can and should start in middle school or high school, especially during the summers. Experience is important for many reasons:

- Shadowing others in the profession can help reveal what the job is really like and whether it's something that you think you want to do, day in and day out. This is a relatively risk-free way to explore different career paths. Ask any seasoned adult and he or she will tell you that figuring out what you *don't* want to do is sometimes more important than figuring out what you *do* want to do.
- Internships and volunteer work are a relatively quick way to gain work experience and develop job skills.
- Volunteering can help you learn the intricacies of the profession, such as what types of environments are best, what kind of care fits you better, and which areas are in more demand.
- Gaining experience during your high school years sets you apart from the many others who are applying to postsecondary programs.
- Volunteering in the field means that you'll be meeting many others doing the job that you might someday want to do (think: career net-

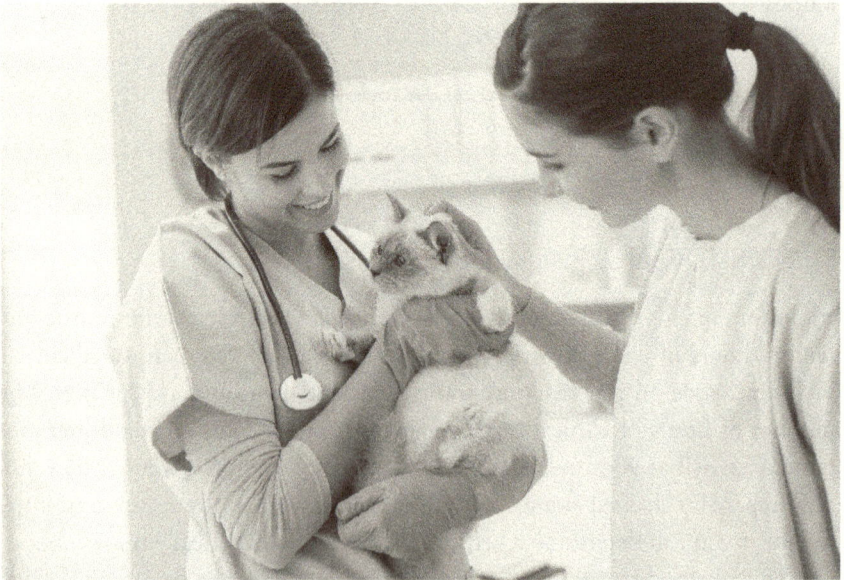

Volunteering in a veterinary setting is just one way to get real-world experience with animals.
©demaerre/iStock/Getty Images

working). You have the potential to develop mentor relationships, culti-vate future job prospects, and get to know people who can recommend you for later positions. Studies show that about 85 percent of jobs are found through personal contacts.[7]

"Start job shadowing, volunteering, or get a part-time job at a kennel so you can see how a practice operates. It's good to see the day-in and day-out of the profession. It's not a profession you should jump into lightly. It's a medical profession, and you need to know what to expect."—Katie Fox, RVT

Experience can come in the form of volunteering at the local vet clinic or animal hospital, taking on an internship in the summer, finding a summer job that complements your interests, or even attending camps that foster your career aspirations. (See the TeenLife site at www.teenlife.com to start.) Con-sider these tidbits of advice to maximize your volunteer experience.[8] They will help you stand out in competitive fields:

- Get diverse experiences. For example, try to shadow in at least two dif-ferent work settings in veterinary care.
- Try to gain forty hours of volunteer experience in each setting. This is typically considered enough to show that you understand what a full workweek looks like in that setting. This can be as few as four to five hours per week over ten weeks or so.
- If your profession has such a job, find an aide/tech position. Working as a paid aide is by far the best experience you can get. This will prepare you nicely for your clinical experiences and tests as well.
- Don't be afraid to ask questions. Just be considerate of the profes-sionals' time and wait until they are not busy to pursue your ques-tions. Asking good questions shows that you have a real curiosity for the profession.
- Maintain and cultivate professional relationships. Write thank-you notes, send updates about your application progress and tell them where you decide to go to school, and check in occasionally. If you want to find a good mentor, you need to be a gracious and willing mentee.

If you're currently in high school and you're seriously thinking about becoming a vet technician, start by reaching out to a vet tech who works at your pet's vet office, or to a family friend who works as a vet tech. Start by asking good questions and showing your curiosity. Ask to shadow them if possible, remembering the guidelines about courtesy above. Don't expect to be paid for any of this effort. The benefit of volunteering is that it's much easier to get your foot in the door, but the drawback is that you typically will not be paid. However, with time and hard work, your volunteer position may turn into something else. Look at these kinds of experiences as ways to learn about the profession, show people how capable you are, and make connections with others that could last your career. It may even help you to get into the program of your choice, and it will definitely help you write your personal statement as to why you want to be a vet tech.

Another way to find a position is to start with your high school guidance counselor or website, visit the websites listed in this book, and search the web for offices in your area. Don't be afraid to pick up the phone and call them. Be prepared to start by cleaning facilities, assisting staff with clerical work, and other such tasks. Being on-site, no matter what you're doing, will teach you more than you know. With a great attitude and work ethic, you will likely be given more responsibility over time. Once you are in your program, you will get many hours of hands-on experience as well.

Networking

Because it's so important, another last word about networking: It's important to develop mentor relationships even at this stage. Remember that about 85 percent of jobs are found through personal contacts. If you know someone in the field, don't hesitate to reach out. Be patient and polite, but ask for help, perspective, and guidance.

If you don't know anyone who is a vet technician, ask your school guidance counselor to help you make connections. Or pick up the phone yourself. Reaching out with a genuine interest in knowledge and a real curiosity about the field will go a long way. You don't need a job or an internship just yet—just a connection that could blossom into a mentoring relationship. Follow these important but simple rules for the best results when networking:

- Do your homework about a potential contact, connection, university, or employer before you make contact. Be sure to have a general understanding of what they do and why. But don't be a know-it-all. Be open and ready to ask good questions.
- Be considerate of professionals' time and resources. Think about what they can get from you in return for mentoring or helping you.
- Speak and write using proper English. Proofread all your letters, e-mails, and even texts. Think about how you will be perceived at all times.
- Always stay positive.

Don't forget that your high school guidance counselor can be a great source of information and connections.

Summary

In this chapter, you learned even more about what it takes to become a vet technician and the various education options you have. You also learned about getting experience in this field before you enter school as well as during the educational process. At this time, you should have a good idea of the educational requirements of the two areas you can pursue. You hopefully even contemplated some questions about what kind of educational career path fits your strengths, time requirements, and wallet. Are you starting to picture your career plan? If not, that's okay, as there's still time.

Remember that no matter which of these roles you pursue, you must maintain licensure and certifications and meet continuing education requirements. Advances in understanding in the fields of health, medicine, nutrition, and more are continuous, and it's vitally important that you keep apprised of what's happening in your field. The bottom line is that you need to have a lifelong love of learning to succeed in any healthcare field, including veterinary medicine.

Chapter 3 goes into a lot more detail about pursuing the best educational path. The chapter covers the process of researching schools and finding the best fit for your needs, as well as how to find the best value for your education, and includes a discussion about financial aid and scholarships. At the end of chapter 3, you should have a much clearer view of the educational landscape and how and where you fit in.

3

Pursuing the Education Path

*W*hen it comes time to start looking at your or postsecondary educational opportunities, many high schoolers tend to freeze up at the enormity of the job ahead of them. This chapter will help break down this process for you so it won't seem so daunting.

It's true that finding the right learning institution is important, and it's a big step toward achieving your career goals and dreams. The last chapter covered the various educational requirements of careers in paraveterinary medicine, which means you should now be ready to find the right institution of learning. This isn't always just a process of finding the very best school that you can afford and can be accepted into, although that might end up being your path. It should also be about finding the right fit so that you can have the best possible experience during your post–high school years.

But here's the truth of it all—attending postsecondary schooling isn't just about getting a degree. It's about learning how to be an adult, managing your life and your responsibilities, being exposed to new experiences, growing as a person, and otherwise moving toward becoming an adult who contributes to society. Postsecondary schooling offers you an opportunity to actually become an interesting person with perspective on the world and empathy and consideration for people other than yourself, if you let it.

An important component of how successful you will be in college is finding the right fit, the right school that brings out the best in you and challenges you at different levels. I know—no pressure, right? Just as with finding the right profession, your ultimate goal should be to match your personal interests, goals, and personality with the college's goals and perspective. For example, small liberal arts colleges have a much different feel and philosophy than Big 10 state schools. And rest assured that all this advice applies even if you're planning on attending community college or another postsecondary school.

Don't worry, though; in addition to these soft skills, this chapter does dive into the nitty-gritty of how to find the best schools, no matter what you want to do. In the healthcare field specifically, attending an accredited program is critical to future success, and that is covered in detail in this chapter.

Finding a School That Fits Your Personality

Before looking at the details of good schools for paraveterinary medicine, it will behoove you to take some time to consider what type of school will be best for you. Answering questions like the ones that follow can help you narrow your search and focus on a smaller set of choices. Write your answers to these questions down somewhere where you can refer to them often, such as in the Notes app on your phone:

- *Size:* Does the size of the school matter to you? Colleges and universities range in size from five hundred or fewer students to forty thousand students.
- *Community location:* Would you prefer to be in a rural area, a small town, a suburban area, or a large city? How important is the location of the school in the larger world?
- *Distance from home:* How far away from home—in terms of hours or miles away—do you want/are you willing to go?
- *Housing options:* What kind of housing would you prefer and can you afford? Dorms, off-campus apartments, and private homes are all common options.
- *Student body:* How would you like the student body to look? Think about coed versus all-male and all-female settings, as well as ethnic and racial makeup, how many students are part-time versus full-time, average age, and the percentage of commuter students.
- *Academic environment:* Which majors are offered, and at which degree levels? Research the student-faculty ratio. Are the classes taught often by actual professors or more often by the teaching assistants? How many internships does the school typically provides to students? Are independent study or study abroad programs available in your area of interest?

- *Financial aid availability/cost:* Does the school provide ample opportunities for scholarships, grants, work-study programs, and the like? Does cost play a role in your options? (For most people, it does.)
- *Support services:* How strong are the school's academic and career placement counseling services?
- *Social activities and athletics:* Does the school offer clubs that you are interested in? Which sports are offered? Are scholarships available?
- *Specialized programs:* Does the school offer honors programs or programs for veterans or students with disabilities or special needs?

Not all of these questions are going to be important to you and that's fine. Be sure to make note of aspects that don't matter as much to you. You might change your mind as you visit colleges, but it's important to make note of where you are to begin with.

U.S. News & World Report puts it best when it reports that the college that fits you best is one that:

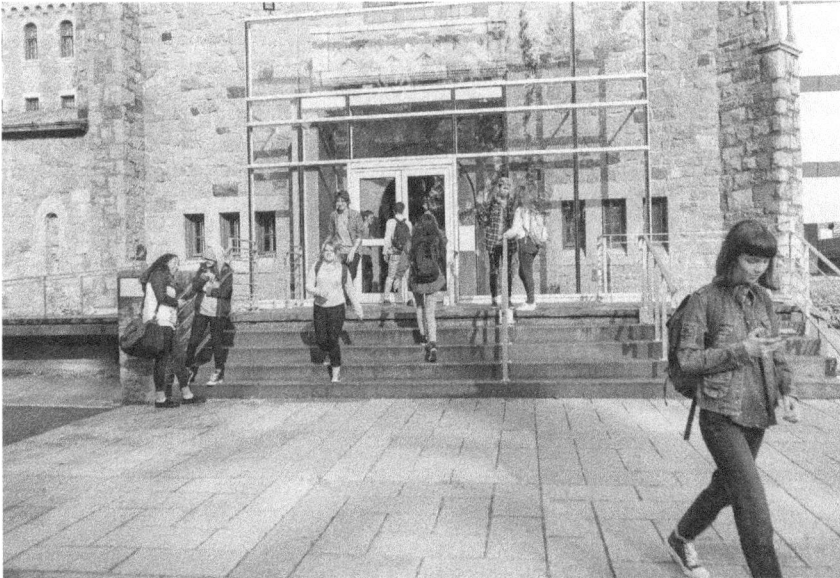

As long as they are accredited, community colleges can be great places of learning for a fraction of the cost. ©*martinedoucet/E+/Getty Images*

- Offers a degree that matches your interests and needs
- Provides a style of instruction that matches the way you like to learn
- Provides a level of academic rigor to match your aptitude and preparation
- Offers a community that feels like home to you
- Values you for what you do well[1]

According to the National Center for Educational Statistics, which is part of the US Department of Education, six years after entering college for an undergraduate degree, only 59 percent of students have graduated.[2] Barely half of those students will graduate from college in their lifetime.[3]

Hopefully, this section has impressed upon you the importance of finding the right educational fit. Take some time to paint a mental picture of the kind of school setting that will best complement your needs.

HOW IMPORTANT IS ACCREDITATION?

Accreditation is the process of ensuring that an academic program meets the common standards of quality set forth for that particular profession. Keep in mind that most companies will hire only people who hold a degree from a program that is accredited. This is especially true in health-related fields such as veterinary medicine, which are more heavily regulated. When you research a school or program, make sure you can verify that the program of study is accredited through the proper accreditation body.

Visit the American Veterinary Medical Association's (AVMA) website at www.avma.org/ProfessionalDevelopment/Education/Accreditation/Programs/Pages/vettech-programs.aspx for an updated and complete list of vet tech programs that have been accredited by the CVTEA, which is the accrediting arm of the AVMA. The site provides links to each state so you can see the accredited programs in your area. This is a good place to start to find a school that's accredited *and* meets your educational and financial needs.

Choosing How to Enter the Field

As you have learned so far in the book, there are different ways you can begin working in paraveterinary medicine. Each of these paths has benefits and drawbacks. Let's look at each a bit more closely.

BEGIN AS A VET ASSISTANT

In theory, you can enter the workforce immediately after high school, without a postsecondary degree, and begin working as a vet assistant. The benefit to this approach is that you can practice in the field without committing too much time and money into it before determining if you really are suited for it. It is the fastest way to enter the profession, although you will most likely need some previous hands-on experience (which you can get by volunteering) if you are entering the field without any schooling.

The drawbacks to this approach are numerous. For one, the profession as a whole is moving toward requiring vet asisstants to be educated and certified. Several states already require this approach. If you did start this way, you will most likely be required to become licensed and continue your education in order to maintain your position. Certainly, if you want to be promoted to positions with more responsibility, you will need to get a degree.

The reality is that others working with you may not give you respect or trust your judgment without a degree or license. They may even resent you, thinking that you did not go through the rigorous process they did to hold a very similar position.

In addition, having a degree confers a certain amount of confidence on its holder that can help in medical siutations. It's not just a piece of paper.

BEGIN AS A VET TECHNICIAN WITH AN ASSOCIATE'S DEGREE

By far the most common way that vet technicians enter the field is by graduating from a two-year American Veterinary Medical Association–accredited program from a community college, college, or university.

After finishing their schooling, technicians usually have to pass an exam and then become registered, licensed, or certified, depending on the requirements in the state in which they work. Vet techs usually have a wider range of responsibilities than vet assistants, often including giving vaccinations, taking blood and inserting catheters, providing emergency care to animals, giving anaesthesia and assisting veterinarians during animal surgeries, and much more. There is currently an initiative to call this profession a veterinary nurse, and you can probably see why.

Vet technicians are generally more respected than vet assistants, and they are given pay and responsibilities commensurate with that respect. However, the drawback is that you need to earn that degree, which can be expensive and time consuming, and maybe even cost-prohibitive for some.

"Getting the associate's degree and being licensed is the biggest difference between an assistant and a credentialed tech. It helps you know why you are doing things. How will it affect the animals and the disease process? Also, most schools have 80–90 percent pass rate on the state and national exams. But not every state requires or recognizes credentialing, which is a huge problem."—Courtney Waxman, RVT

BEGIN AS A VET TECHNOLOGIST WITH A BACHELOR'S DEGREE

Veterinary technologists are graduates from a four-year AVMA-accredited bachelor's degree program. Many work in more advanced research-related jobs or laboratory settings, usually under the guidance of a scientist or a veterinarian, but they also can and do work as vet technicians in animal clinics and hospitals.

The bottom line is that in most cases, having a bachelor's degree doesn't set you apart from those who hold an associate's degree. Recall from chapter 1 that at this time, very few states recognize the title of veterinary technologist, and in all the rest, the credential granted is licensed/registered/certified veterinary technician regardless of whether the person has an associate's degree or a bachelor's degree.[4] That means your debt-to-income ratio could be twice that as a vet technician. This refers to the amount of debt someone has due to student loans compared to their potential income.

It's possible to earn a higher salary with the bachelor's degree if you choose the right type of career—research, teaching, working for drug companies, working in a specialty practice, and so on. But it's just as common that you will make the same money as any other veterinary technician, at least until you prove yourself to be a more valuable asset.

Researching Schools

If you're currently in high school and you are serious about pursuing a career as a vet technician or technologist, whether by earning an associate's degree or a bachelor's degree, start by finding four to five schools in a realistic location (for you) that offer the degree, certificate, or program you want to pursue. Not every school near you or that you have an initial interest in will offer the program you want, of course, so narrow your choices accordingly. With that said, consider attending a university in your resident state, if possible; this will save you lots of money. Private institutions don't typically discount resident student tuition costs.

Be sure you research the basic grade point average (GPA) and SAT or ACT requirements of each school as well.

For students applying to associate's degree programs or greater, most advisers recommend that students take both the ACT and the SAT during the spring of their junior year at the latest. (The ACT test is generally considered more heavily weighted in science, so it may be more important for you.) You can retake these tests and use your highest score, so be sure to leave time for a retake early in your senior year if needed. You want your best score to be available to all the schools you're applying to by January of your senior year, which will also enable your score to be considered with any scholarship applications. Keep in mind these are general timelines—be sure to check the exact deadlines and calendars of the schools to which you're applying!

Once you have found four to five accredited schools in a realistic location for you that offer the degree or certificate you are looking for, spend some time on their websites studying the requirements for admissions. Most schools will list the average stats for the last class accepted to each program. Important factors in your decision about what schools to apply to should include whether or not you meet the requirements, your chances of getting in (but shoot high!), tuition costs and availability of scholarships and grants, location, and the school's reputation and licensure/graduation rates. And of course, make sure the schools you are considering are accredited.

The importance of these characteristics will depend on your grades and test scores, your financial resources, and other personal factors. You of course want to find a university that has a good reputation for the science, biology, and veterinary medicine fields, but it's also important to match your academic rigor and practical needs with the best school you can.

SARAH JO BOULDIN

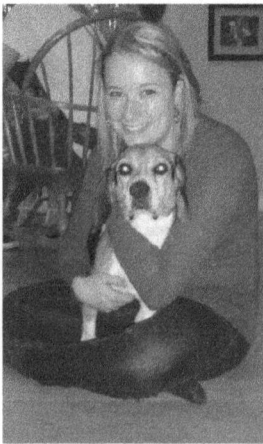

Sarah Jo Bouldin.
Courtesy of Sarah Jo Bouldin

Sarah Jo Bouldin started the vet technology program in 2012 and graduated in 2014. That fall, she got her license to practice in North Carolina and got a job at the animal hospital about three months before she graduated. She has worked there ever since. She is just now reaching her five-year mark!

When she started there, the hospital had three doctors, and she worked her way up to the head of surgery and treatment. She is a registered veterinary technician (RVT) and does everything short of surgery and prescribing medicine.

Can you explain how you became interested in becoming a vet technician?

As long as I can remember, I wanted to be a vet! I would take care of my dog stuffed animals and cut them open and then sew them back up. I pulled ticks off our dogs!

The older I got, the more I realized what a vet did. But what I wanted was to be with the animals and care for them—essentially be a "vet nurse." I thought of getting a degree in animal science, but they didn't do what I wanted to do. Instead, that's a stepping-stone maybe to vet school. You can't become an RVT with an animal science degree. That wasn't the career I wanted to do. I didn't know that RVT was a job! My mom found it out and told me about it. So I got my degree!

Can you describe what you do in your daily job?

As I mentioned, I can do everything short of surgery and prescribing medicine. I take care of patients, draw blood, run blood work, take care of hospitalized pets, place IV catheters, take radiographs, intubate patients, monitor them while they are under anesthesia, recover them from surgery, dental cleanings, nail trims, wound dressing—pretty much everything all over the board!

You still have to work with owners and have people skills. You need to help the owners feel better, feel safe, comfortable, etc. Owner/client education is a little less than 50 percent of the job! I might do more than others, because I like it. I do enjoy working with owners.

What's the best part of your job?

My favorite part is helping animals feel better. When they wake up from surgery and they are sad and scared and hurt, I can comfort them and make the pain go away and calm them. I often sing to them too when they are coming out of sedation. I also love making the owners feel better too.

At the end of the day, seeing a sick pet feel better is so rewarding! So sick they can't move and then two days later, they walk out wagging their tail. It's very cool to see how medicine works and turn a life around.

One of my favorite phrases is—"I'm not in it for the income, I am in it for the outcome!"

What's the most challenging part of your job?

Having to say goodbye! It's tough to say goodbye to a pet you've gotten to know and seen over time. Most of the time, it's the right decision. Doing this because of behavioral issues is really hard, even though it might be right. It's comforting because you know they are no longer in pain. Dealing with the end of life is very tough.

Do you think education prepared you for your job?

Yes, and I hated school. I was a C student in high school. Then I graduated with honors in this program. It really turned me around about schooling. I learned the most right after I graduated and applied what I learned to real-life circumstances. When you are in actual circumstances and apply what you learned in the classroom, you really learn it well then.

Studying for the boards and working in the practice was a great education. The forty hours of volunteer work that I did at a local animal hospital before applying to the program was also a great education.

Do you recommend to others that they get the RVT license?

Yes. RVTs are licensed. Animal care assistants aren't licensed, so in North Carolina, they can't give vaccines and other critical care. But we teach a lot in the hospital. A lot of them want to be RVTs or vets, so they are given the opportunity to learn. Many hospitals don't have RVTs but just have people who have learned on the job. They don't have to pay people without a license as much. Clinics don't pay assistants as much.

Ask if your vet uses RVTs. If they are monitoring anesthesia and something bad happens, that's bad. You want someone qualified to monitor your pet. They will be in better hands. We do have the knowledge to do a superior job.

What are some things in this profession that are especially challenging right now?

One of the biggest things is the turnover in the profession. I had thirty-seven graduate in my class five years ago and there are now less than twenty still practicing. It's because they are underappreciated and underpaid. We aren't recognized as we should be. People don't appreciate what an RVT is and does.

What are some characteristics of a good vet tech?

Compassion and empathy for pets *and* owners are very important. Technical skills are very important too, of course. People skills are important. You have to be on your toes. You can't make mistakes because lives are on the line. This is someone's "child." Millennials will go into debt for their pets! This could be someone's baby. Take your time with every pet.

Also, you can't be judgmental about people's decisions regarding their pets. This is one of my biggest pet peeves. You don't know what they are going through. This is a huge red flag for me.

What advice do you have for young people considering this career?

Make sure it's what you want to do. Realize it's not just about animals. It's about people too. If you "hate" people, it's probably not for you. It's a big commitment. You're not going to be rich. I am appreciated where I work, but that's not always the case. There are vet clinics who do appreciate RVTs and understand the value of the job. It is rewarding and possible to love it. Be educated about the position.

How can a young person prepare for a career as a vet technician while in high school?

Research the schools and the requirements and get them done ahead of time. Have some background working in an animal hospital or volunteering. This will give you a huge leg up during school. Do the research. Get a job in a vet clinic.

Any last thoughts?

I love what I do. I wouldn't change it for the world. I feel appreciated where I am. You can find that too, with some work. It's rewarding. I could not imagine doing anything else.

THE MOST PERSONAL OF PERSONAL STATEMENTS

The personal statement you include with your application to college is extremely important, especially if your GPA and SAT/ACT scores are on the border of what is typically accepted. Write something that is thoughtful and conveys your understanding of the paraveterinary medicine profession, as well as your desire to practice in this field. Why are you uniquely qualified? Why are you a good fit for the school or program? These essays should be highly personal (the "personal" in personal statement). Will the admissions professionals who read it—along with hundreds of others—come away with a snapshot of who you really are and what you are passionate about?

Look online for some examples of good personal statements, which will give you a feel for what works. Be sure to check your specific school for length guidelines, format requirements, and any other guidelines they expect you to follow.

And of course, be sure to proofread it several times and ask a professional (such as your school writing center or your local library services) to proofread it as well.

What's It Going to Cost You?

So, the bottom line: What will your education end up costing you? Of course, this depends on many factors, including the type and length of degree you pursue, where you attend (in-state or not, private or public institution), how much in scholarships or financial aid you're able to obtain, your family or personal income, and many other factors. The National Center for Education Statistics tracks and summarizes financial data from colleges and universities all over the

United States. (You can find more information at http://nces.ed.gov.) A sample of the most recent data is shown in Table 3.1.

Table 3.1.   Average Yearly Tuition, Fees, Room, and Board for Full-Time Undergraduates[5]

Year	Public 4-Year, In-State	Public 4-Year, Out-of-State	Private Nonprofit
2016–2017	$19,488	Not available	$41,465
2017–2018	$20,050	$25,657	$43,139

Source: National Center for Education Statistics, nces.ed.gov

Keep in mind these are averages and reflect the published prices, not the net prices. If you read data about a particular university or find averages in your particular area of interest, you should assume those numbers are closer to reality than these, as they are more specific. This data helps to show you the ballpark figures. The College Board website (www.collegeboard.org) also has pertinent statistics.

Another way to look at it is that earning a two-year associate's degree costs about $25,000 to $30,000. You can expect to pay about half that for a one-year nondegree certificate.

> The actual, final price (or net price) that you'll pay for a specific college is the published price (tuition and fees) to attend that college, minus any grants, scholarships, and education tax benefits you receive. This difference can be significant. According to the College Board, "in 2015–2016, the average published price of in-state tuition and fees for public four-year colleges was about $9,410. But the average net price of in-state tuition and fees for public four-year colleges was only about $3,980."[6]

Generally speaking, there is about a 3 percent annual increase in tuition and associated costs to attend college. In other words, if you are expecting to attend college two years after this data was collected, you need to add approximately 6 percent to these numbers. Keep in mind that this assumes no financial aid or scholarships of any kind.

This chapter discusses finding the most affordable path to get the degree you want. Later in this chapter, you'll also learn how to prime the pumps and get as much money for college as you can.

WHAT IS A GAP YEAR?

Taking a year off between high school and college, often called a gap year, is normal, perfectly acceptable, and almost required in many countries around the world. It is becoming increasingly acceptable in the United States as well. Even Malia Obama, President Obama's daughter, did it. Because the cost of college has gone up dramatically, it literally pays for you to know going in what you want to study, and a gap year—well spent—can do lots to help you answer that question.

Some great ways to spend your gap year include joining organizations such as the Peace Corps or AmeriCorps, enrolling in a mountaineering program or other gap year–styled program, backpacking across Europe or other countries on the cheap (be safe and bring a friend), finding a volunteer organization that furthers a cause you believe in or that complements your career aspirations, joining a Road Scholar program (see www.roadscholar.org), teaching English in another country (see www .gooverseas.com/blog/best-countries-for-seniors-to-teach-english-abroad for more information), or working and earning money for college!

Many students will find that they get much more out of college when they have a year to mature and to experience the real world. The American Gap Year Association reports from alumni surveys that students who take gap years show increased civic engagement, higher college graduation rates, and improved GPAs in college.[7]

See the association's website at https://gapyearassociation.org for lots of advice and resources if you're considering this potentially life-altering experience.

Making the Most of School Visits

If it's at all practical and feasible, you should visit the schools you're considering. To get a real feel for any college or school, you need to walk around the campus and buildings, spend some time in the common areas where students hang out, and sit in on a few classes. You can also sign up for campus tours, which are typically given by current students. This is another good way to see the school and ask questions of someone who knows. Be sure to visit the specific school/building that covers your intended major as well. Websites and brochures won't be able to convey that intangible feeling you'll get from a visit.

Make a list of questions that are important to you before you visit. In addition to the questions listed earlier in this chapter, consider these questions as well:

- What is the makeup of the current freshman class? Is the campus diverse?
- What is the meal plan like? What are the food options?
- Where do most of the students hang out between classes? (Be sure to visit this area.)
- How long does it take to walk from one end of the campus to the other?
- What types of transportation are available for students? Does campus security provide escorts to cars, dorms, and other on-campus destinations at night?

To prepare for your visit and make the most of it, consider these tips and words of advice:

- Be sure to do some research. At the very least, spend some time on the college's website. You may find your questions are addressed adequately there.
- Make a list of questions.
- Arrange to meet with a professor in your area of interest or to visit the specific school.
- Be prepared to answer questions about yourself and why you are interested in this school.
- Dress in neat, clean, and casual clothes. Avoid overly wrinkled clothing or anything with stains.

Finally, be sure to send thank-you notes or e-mails after the visit is over. Remind recipients of when you visited the campus and thank them for their time.

Financial Aid and Student Loans

Finding the money to attend college—whether a two- or four-year college program, an online program, or a vocational career college—can seem overwhelming. But you can do it if you have a plan before you actually start applying to colleges. If you get into your top-choice university, don't let the sticker price

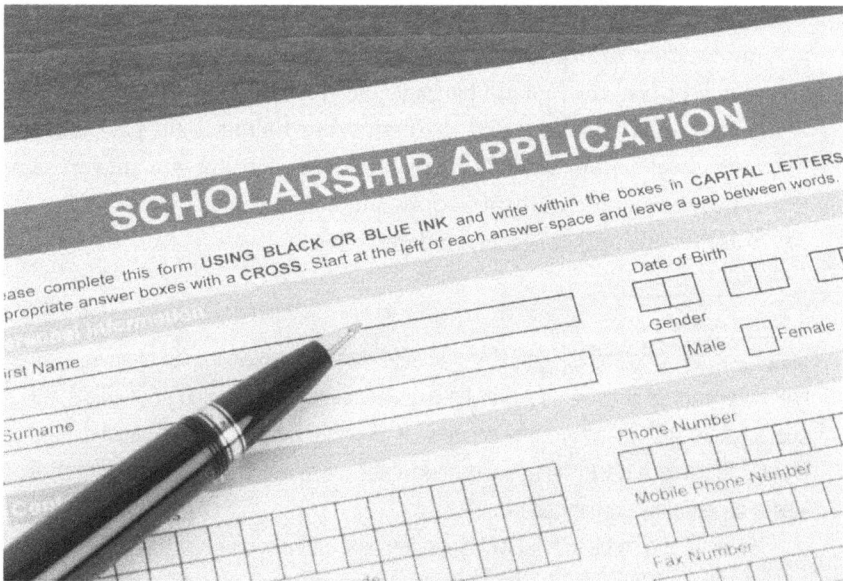

Paying for college can take a creative mix of grants, scholarships, and loans, but you can find your way with some help! ©Casper1774Studio/iStock/Getty Images

turn you away. Financial aid can come from many different sources, and it's available to cover all different kinds of costs you'll encounter during your years in college, including tuition, fees, books, housing, and food.

The good news is that universities more often offer incentive or tuition discount aid to encourage students to attend. The market is often more competitive in the favor of the student, and colleges and universities are responding by offering more generous aid packages to a wider range of students than they used to. Here are some basic tips and pointers about the financial aid process:

- Apply for financial aid during your senior year. You must fill out the Free Application for Federal Student Aid (FAFSA) form, which can be filed starting October 1 of your senior year until June of the year you graduate.[8] Because the amount of available aid is limited, it's best to apply as soon as you possibly can. See https://studentaid.ed.gov/sa/fafsa to get started.
- Be sure to compare and contrast the deals you get at different schools. There is room to negotiate with universities. The first offer for aid may not be the best you'll get.

- Wait until you receive all offers from your top schools and then use this information to negotiate with your top choice to see if the school will match or beat the best aid package you received.
- To be eligible to keep and maintain your financial aid package, you must meet certain grade/GPA requirements. Be sure you are very clear about these academic expectations and keep up with them.
- You must reapply for federal aid every year.

Watch out for scholarship scams! You should never be asked to pay to submit the FAFSA form (*free* is in its name) or be required to pay a lot to find appropriate aid and scholarships. These are free services. If an organization promises you'll get aid or says that you have to "act now or miss out," these are both warning signs of a less-than-reputable organization.

You should also be careful with your personal information to avoid identity theft as well. Simple things like closing and exiting your browser after visiting sites where you entered personal information goes a long way. Don't share your student aid ID number with anyone, either.

It's important to understand the different forms of financial aid that are available to you. That way, you'll know how to apply for different kinds and get the best financial aid package that fits your needs and strengths. The two main categories that financial aid falls under is gift aid, which doesn't have to be repaid, and self-help aid, which includes loans that must be repaid and work-study funds that are earned. The next sections cover the various types of financial aid that fit into these areas.

GRANTS

Grants typically are awarded to students who have financial need, but can also be used in the areas of athletics, academics, demographics, veteran support, and special talents. They do not have to be paid back. Grants can come from federal agencies, state agencies, specific universities, and private organizations. Most federal and state grants are based on financial need.

SCHOLARSHIPS

Scholarships are merit-based aid that does not have to be paid back. They are typically awarded based on academic excellence or some other special talent, such as music or art. Scholarships can also be athletic-based, minority-based, aid for women, and so forth. These are typically not awarded by federal or state governments, but instead come from the specific school you applied to as well as private and nonprofit organizations.

Be sure to reach out directly to the financial aid officers of the schools you want to attend. These people are great contacts who can lead you to many more sources of scholarships and financial aid. Visit GoCollege's Financial Aid Finder at www.gocollege.com/financial-aid/scholarships/types for lots more information about how scholarships in general work.

LOANS

Many types of loans are available especially for students to pay for their post-secondary education. However, the important thing to remember here is that loans must be paid back, with interest. (This is the extra cost of borrowing the money and is usually a percentage of the amount you borrow.) Be sure you understand the interest rate you will be charged. Is this fixed or will it change over time? Are payments on the loan and interest deferred until you graduate (meaning you don't have to begin paying it off until after you graduate)? Is the loan subsidized (meaning the federal government pays the interest until you graduate)? These are all points you need to be clear about before you sign on the dotted line.

There are many types of loans offered to students, including need-based loans, non-need-based loans, state loans, and private loans. Two very reputable federal loans are the Perkins Loan and the Direct Stafford Loan. For more information about student loans, visit https://bigfuture.collegeboard.org/pay -for-college/loans/types-of-college-loans.

FEDERAL WORK-STUDY

The US federal work-study program provides part-time jobs for undergraduate and graduate students with financial need so they can earn money to pay for educational expenses. The focus of such work is on community service work and work related to a student's course of study. Not all schools participate in this program, so be sure to check with the financial aid office at any schools you are considering if this is something you are counting on. The sooner you apply, the more likely you will get the job you desire and be able to benefit from the program, as funds are limited. See https://studentaid.ed.gov/sa/types/work -study for more information about this opportunity.

JIA WANG

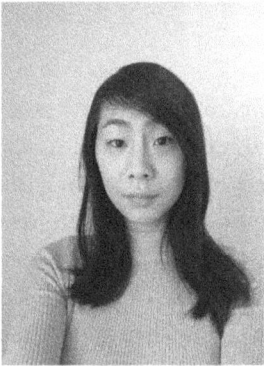

Jia Wang.
Courtesy of Jia Wang

Jia Wang graduated in 2018 with her vet technology degree. She started in the field at the young age of seventeen as a kennel attendant and worked her way up. She became a registered vet technician in 2018 and currently works as an RVT at an animal hospital. She wants to continue her education to become a veterinary pathologist.

Can you explain how you became interested in becoming a vet technician?

I always knew that I wanted to work with animals even though I didn't know much about the veterinary field. When I was young, we had a negative experience at a vet with our family dog. I knew that something had to change, and I wanted to contribute to that change. It was a cold, not a kind experience. I wanted it to be welcoming. Healthcare should be comfort- and patient-focused.

Can you talk about your current position? What's a typical day in your job?

I do a little bit of everything at the animal hospital. We have different zones—X-rays, blood work, wellness, and surgery, for example.

When I work in the surgery zone, I set up for the surgery, follow the protocol, and get the flow from the doctor. I get the meds prepared and place the catheter. Surgeries usually take several hours, so by noon they are done. At that point, I write notes and make sure the animals are recovering okay and then educate owners about taking the pets home. I also tell the owners what happened to their pets.

Do you think your education prepared you for your job? Do you recommend getting the RVT license?

My education gave me a good foundation. A lot of the learning is through practice and applying the skills to actual animals. You don't get to practice as much in school. Applying skills is so important!

Yes, get the license—it helps you know how to handle many difficult situations and it gives you confidence. You can handle situations more efficiently and give better patient care.

What's the best part of being a vet technician?

I love seeing the difference we make. Helping fearful or injured patients feel better. When owners acknowledge that, it's especially nice. It's great when the animals are better and wagging their tails and I contributed to that.

How can people avoid burnout in this job?

Separate your work from your personal life. It's good to be caring and empathetic, but you can't carry those burdens home. Having a good routine for self-care is very important, as it helps relieve emotional stress.

What are some things in this profession that are especially challenging right now?

One of my biggest things that I am passionate about is the fear-free movement! When you are given more room and time to work with patients, in the long run, it is better. There is short-term resistance from some owners and doctors because it takes more time.

What are some characteristics of a good vet technician?

You must be patient and diligent and be able to handle a heavy workload and multitask. You have to be able to pace yourself.

What is the most surprising thing about your job? Is it what you expected it would be?

The tough cases where the patient does not have a happy ending. That sticks with you. It's hard to get over. I remember all the names.

Some parts are unexpected because, until you get in there and work, you really don't know what to expect. The day-to-day can be challenging.

Where do you see yourself going from here? Where do you see the field going from here?

I am currently working on my undergrad education—I want to finish in two and a half years and then start veterinary school in about three years. There are four years of vet school and then a three-year residency in pathology. In vet tech school, we talked about cellular changes and I thought it was so interesting that each disease process has its own path—under a microscope you can see that. It blew my mind.

The field is on an upward trend. I'd like to see a greater difference between the vet assistant and the vet technician. There *is* a difference in requirements. Or maybe call them veterinary nurses. In either case, I want that vet tech title/role to be acknowledged and get better pay.

Veterinary assistants don't always need an education—you can get certified. It has a much smaller scale in terms of education and a lot of people don't recognize it.

What advice do you have for young people considering this career?

Get an early start. Right out of high school or during high school. It really helped me and gave me insight into the career field. Early exposure helps with that.

I wish I had known even earlier that the veterinary technician was an actual position. Not all people know this. I went through bumps to find this actual path. I want people to know that there is something in the field other than being a veterinarian.

How can a young person prepare for a career as a vet technician while in high school?

Reach out to places around you—clinics, humane shelters, rescue organizations, etc. Even if you could just be a receptionist or kennel assistant. Be proactive about getting your foot in the door.

Humane societies are not bad at all, but you'll see sadder cases and it can be hard to see pets euthanized and such. It can be hard to take. The chance for emotional burnout is greater here.

Making High School Count

If you are still in high school or middle school, there are still many things you can do now to help the postsecondary educational process go more smoothly. Consider these tips for your remaining years:

- Work on listening well and speaking and communicating clearly. Work on writing clearly and effectively.

- Learn how to learn. This means keeping an open mind, asking questions, asking for help when you need it, taking good notes, and doing your homework.
- Plan a daily homework schedule and keep up with it. Have a consistent, quiet place to study.
- Talk about your career interests with friends, family, and counselors. They may have connections to people in your community whom you can shadow or who will mentor you.
- Try new interests and activities, especially during your first two years of high school.
- Be involved in extracurricular activities that truly interest you and say something about who you are and who you want to be. This probably means you need to work with animals in as many settings as you can!

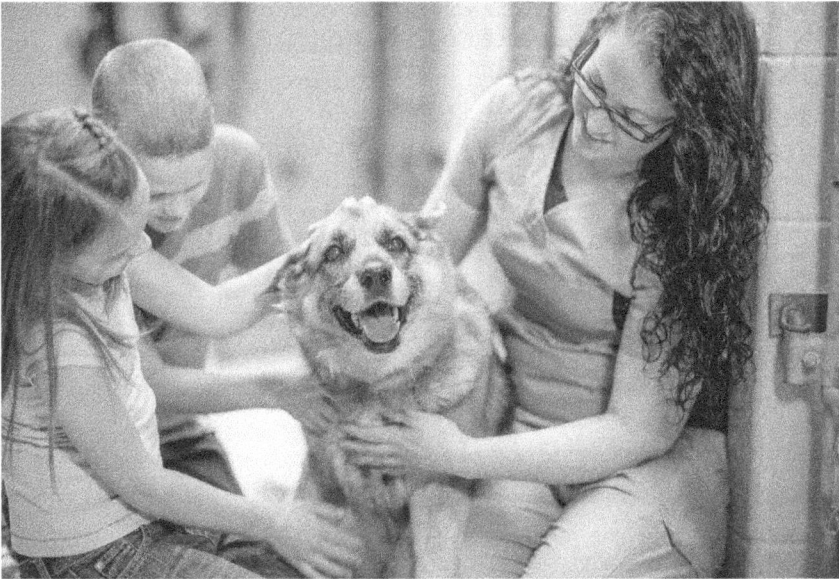

Volunteering is a great way to get résumé-worthy experience and find out if you really love the job.
©FatCamera/E+/Getty Images

KATIE FOX

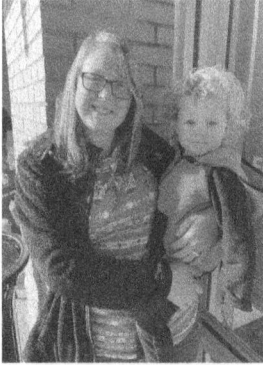

Katie Fox earned her associate's degree in 2015 as a veterinary technician and then became credentialed as an RVT. She started her career in 2012 as an assistant at a clinic where she had volunteered in high school. She worked there until graduating from college in 2015. She then worked at a mixed-practice clinic (which cares for large and small animals) until 2017, when she took time off for her baby. She then worked in an emergency hospital setting for one and a half years. In July 2019, she started full-time at a private practice animal clinic.

Can you explain how you became interested in becoming a vet technician?

I lived out in the country and worked on the farm growing up. We worked with our large-animal vet and did a lot. The large-animal vet taught us how to give injections and other procedures. It sparked my interest in helping animals, day in and day out, on the farm. Then in high school I volunteered at a clinic.

I was also heavily involved in 4-H growing up. I showed dairy cows, dairy steer, beef cows, and horses and pigs too. I got a lot of hands-on skills that way.

What's the best part of your job?

Getting to see super-sick animals recover and spend more years with their families is very rewarding. Seeing the recovery and helping the animals that no one wants.

What's the most challenging part of your job?

I guess I would say noncompliant owners and owners who think they can't do any-thing because of money, which leads to animals suffering. That's never something you want to see. For example, we might see puppies that have parvo and owners can't afford the treatment. So puppies suffer and die. That's hard to watch.

Do you think your education prepared you for your job?

I was working at a clinic while going to school, which was the best combination. I could practice what I was learning at school. The hands-on experience is really important, because it's a hands-on field. I am licensed, but you don't have to be in Indiana. There are some things that nonlicensed people can't do.

If you're able to do it, work somewhere while going to school. Even volunteering or shadowing is very helpful. It can help you make sure it's the right field for you.

Your knowledge and abilities include a wide range of all different kinds of animals. It's trickier to know normal ranges and doses for all kinds of pets. The wide variety of knowledge can be nice too. ER especially is challenging, but in a good way too.

What are some things in this profession that are especially challenging right now?

The way that they are changing the controlled substances and logging them all in. I understand it, but it makes it harder to get everything done in a busy day. Also, parvo outbreaks have been bad this year, and it's hard to see a puppy die just because of that. We see parvo coming right from the breeders.

Also, vet techs often aren't treated as well as nurses. There aren't respected as much. That affects salaries, health insurance, and more. People don't see it as a medical profession.

What are some characteristics of a good vet technician?

Attention to detail, good teamwork and communication skills, and honesty. Hard worker.

You still have to deal with owners and be able to work with people. You need to work with people and find the balance in helping the owners and helping the pets, and sometimes those issues are at odds.

How do you avoid burnout?

Find hobbies and things outside the field that you enjoy. Look at the positive cases too. When you have a rough day, you have to find the positives in what you do.

What advice do you have for young people considering this career?

Start job shadowing, volunteering, or get a part-time job at a kennel so you can see how a practice operates. It's good to see the day-in and day-out of the profession. It's not a profession you should jump into lightly. It's a medical profession, and you need to know what to expect.

You do have fun snuggling with cats and dogs, but you also see sick animals whom you can't snuggle with. You place an IV and get blood and they don't know what's happening. You look like the bad guy to those animals and you have to be okay with that.

Have there been unexpected/surprising things you've found during your career?

I knew what to expect because I worked in it. Clinics all do things differently and none is wrong per se, but you need to be ready to work with all different styles and approaches.

How can a young person prepare for a career as a vet technician while in high school?

Job shadowing or volunteering. You need a love for animals and good people skills.

Any last thoughts?

It's a great field, but it's not for everybody. It's rewarding more than it is upsetting. But you do have rough patches. Look for the positives! Keep yourself in a positive headspace.

———————

Kids are under so much pressure these days to do it all, but you should think about working smarter rather than harder. If you are involved in things you enjoy, your educational load won't seem like such a burden. Be sure to take time for self-care, such as sleep, unscheduled downtime, and activities that you find fun and energizing. See chapter 4 for more ways to relieve and avoid stress.

Summary

This chapter looked at all the aspects of college and postsecondary schooling that you'll want to consider as you move forward. Remember that finding the right fit is especially important, as it increases the chances that you'll stay in school and finish your degree or program—and have an amazing experience while you're there. The careers covered in this book have varying educational requirements, which means that finding the right school depends a great deal on your career aspirations.

In this chapter, you learned about how to find a good educational fit and how to get the best education for the best deal. You also learned a little about scholarships and financial aid, how the SAT and ACT work, and how to write a unique personal statement that eloquently expresses your passions.

Use this chapter as a jumping-off point to dig deeper into your particular area of interest, but don't forget these important points:

- Take the SAT and ACT early in your junior year so you have time to take them again if you need to. Most schools automatically accept the highest scores.

- Make sure that the school you plan to attend has an accredited program in your field of study. This is particularly important in the veterinary medicine field. Some professions follow national accreditation policies, while others are state-mandated and therefore differ across state lines. Do your research and understand the differences.
- Your personal statement is a very important piece of your application that can set you apart from other applicants. Take the time and energy needed to make it unique and compelling.
- Don't assume you can't afford a school based on the sticker price. Many schools offer great scholarships and aid to qualified students. It doesn't hurt to apply. This advice especially applies to minorities, veterans, and students with disabilities.
- Don't lose sight of the fact that it's important to pursue a career that you enjoy, are good at, and are passionate about! You'll be a happier person if you do so.

At this point, your career goals and aspirations should be gelling. At the very least, you should have a plan for finding out more information. And don't forget about networking, which was covered in more detail in chapter 2.

Chapter 4 goes into detail about the next steps—writing a résumé and cover letter, interviewing well, follow-up communications, and more. This information is not just for college grads; you can use it to secure internships, volunteer positions, summer jobs, and more. In fact, the sooner you can hone these communication skills, the better off you'll be in the professional world.

4

Writing Your Résumé and Interviewing

No matter which path you decide to take—whether you enter the workforce immediately after high school, go to college first and then find yourself looking for a job, or maybe do something in between—having a well-written résumé and impeccable interviewing skills will help you reach your ultimate goals. This chapter provides some helpful tips and advice to build the best résumé and cover letter, how to interview well with prospective employers, and how to communicate effectively and professionally at all times. The advice in this chapter isn't just for people entering the workforce full-time, either; it can help you score that internship or summer job or help you give a great college interview to impress the admissions office.

After discussing how to write your résumé, the chapter looks at important interviewing skills that you can build and develop over time. The chapter also has some tips for dealing successfully with stress, which is an inevitable by-product of a busy life.

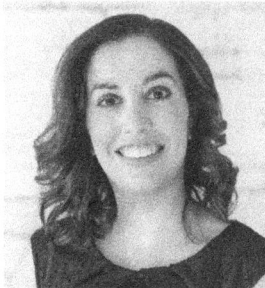

Courtney Waxman.
Courtesy of Courtney Waxman

COURTNEY WAXMAN

Courtney Waxman graduated in 2008 with an associate of applied science in vet technology in Arizona. She became a credentialed veterinary technician after taking the national and state exams. She worked twelve or thirteen years in private emergency and specialty practice in the Phoenix area. In 2017 she got her advanced credential of a veterinary technician specialist in ER and critical care.

In 2018 she moved to Indiana, then went through state process again to be an RVT. She currently works at Purdue University as an instructor for its veterinary nursing program. She also works per diem shifts at Purdue's vet teaching hospital to keep her skills and knowledge fresh.

Can you explain how you became interested in this career path?

Since I was a kid, I wanted to work with animals. Since elementary school, really. During my freshman and sophomore years, I thought I wanted to be a veterinarian at a small practice. My junior year in high school, I looked into the schooling and I realized it was highly competitive—there are only thirty-two colleges in the country (compared to hundreds of human medical schools in the United States). The admissions requirements and courses were rigorous, and many had one- to two-year waiting lists. So I looked into other careers that were similar and found out about vet technicians.

In my last years of high school, I took a job at a general practice where my family took our pets. Once I started working alongside the vet techs, I fully understood all that they did and I realized that I wanted to do what they did.

What's the best part of being a vet technician?

How involved you are with patient care. You provide a ton of nursing care to these animals. I work in critical care, and you can really care for them and nurse them back to health. You do much of the hands-on tasks, rather than the vet. You are highly involved, which is very rewarding.

What's the most challenging part of being a vet technician, in your opinion?

Not being recognized or utilized for my knowledge and skill set. If you're working in a practice where you can't use your skills and degree, that's frustrating.

Why does this happen? Vets aren't always educated about what vet techs do. Of the thirty-two vet schools, only three have a program for vet techs too. Purdue is one. You work, train, and learn alongside each other and understand what each other does.

Some vet techs don't know the difference between credentialed and not. Some field areas don't recognize the specialty areas. These are all issues we need to address through education.

Do you think the education adequately prepares vet technicians to do the job?

Absolutely! That's the biggest difference between an assistant and a credentialed tech. Why you are doing this? How will it affect the animals and the disease process? Understanding the why behind what you are doing is important to growth and excelling in this field.

Most schools have 80–90 percent pass rate on the state and national exams to get credentialed as well. But not every state requires or recognizes credentialing, which is a huge problem.

What are some things in this profession that are especially challenging right now?

There is a national shortage of vets and vet techs. The average length of a vet tech career is about five to six years. Also, as I mentioned, credentialing is not a requirement and not required in every state. Literally anyone off the street can walk into a facility and could be trained on the job and be called a vet tech assistant or even a technician, because it's not regulated.

The vet nurse initiative is to develop one national, unified title so that it is the same in all states. The veterinary nurse title would give us title protection, where uncredentialed assistants couldn't legally use the term without legal consequences. It would have a defined scope of practice also, so every state would know what vet nurses can and can't do. The national title and scope of practice would lead to better job fulfillment, better wages, better use of the nurse, better recognition of the job by clients, and so on.

We have been working three to four years to make this happen, and there is active legislation in three or four states. It's a slow process. This initiative started in 2014–2015 and we are making progress. You can call yourself a vet nurse, so some places are trying to adopt that nomenclature. Purdue, for example, is changing the program and degree to vet nursing. The idea is to have a title commensurate with our skills and schooling. Nursing is what we do with animals.

Other issues include a lack of public recognition about this role, low wages, burnout, and compassion fatigue. Debt-to-income ratio is high in this profession. The suicide rate is very high for vets and (lesser so for) vet techs.

What are some characteristics of a good vet technician?

You should be eager to learn. It's a lifelong-learning career that's always evolving and changing. You need to be flexible and be a multitasker. You must be organized and prioritize what needs to happen first. You should also be caring and compassionate. You need to develop good communication skills with owners, the docs, and your team. Be ready for anything, especially when you're working in the ER. Don't be afraid to ask lots of questions—it's okay if you don't know something. Use it as a learning opportunity.

How can a vet technician avoid burnout and compassion fatigue?

Burnout is an exhaustion of the workplace—you are overworked, have too much overtime, work undesirable shifts, are bullied, aren't utilized, see too much negativity, and so on. In that case, find a workplace that recognizes credentialed people, utilizes you to your full potential, and supports your desire to go to school—one that has a great team culture and atmosphere.

Compassion fatigue is related to your love of animals and you just see too much awfulness. Lots of euthanasia, animal hoarding, dogfighting situations, poor owners, etc. In that case, self-care is very important. Talk to a professional if needed. Turn off work and set healthy boundaries when you're not at work, especially with clients. Work with a good team that's supportive. Have a self-care day or mental health day without guilt. A boundary between work and the rest of your life is important!

What advice do you have for young people considering this career?

Do your research. I see lots of confusion because some people think that becoming a vet tech is a step toward becoming a vet. That's not really true. Figure out what you ultimately want to do. Talk to vet clinics that are local to your area about shadowing, volunteering, or being mentored by them.

Handling animals in a medical setting is a lot different than just liking animals. You see animals euthanized. You need a strong science background too. What you see when visiting your vet office is only a little slice of the job. It's not all sunshine and happiness.

How can a young person prepare for a career as a vet technician while in high school?

Talk to your family veterinarian about different options that are in your local area. The FFA (Future Farmers of America) is a big resource in Indiana, for example. Purdue does agriculture and livestock health. Also talk with advisers—high school, local area, colleges, etc. Of course, talk to vets or vet techs and start there.

Any closing comments?

I still learn something new every day and I am almost fifteen years in. That's one of the best things. You are always learning!

Writing Your Résumé

If you're a teen writing a résumé for your first job, you likely don't have a lot of work experience under your belt yet. Because of this limited work experience, you need to include classes and coursework that are related to the job you're seeking, as well as any school activities and volunteer experience you have. While you are writing your résumé, you might discover some talents and recall some activities you did that you forgot about but that are important to add. Think about volunteer work, side jobs you've held—especially when they are relevant (dog walking, cat sitting, etc.)—and the like. A good approach at this point in your career is to build a functional résumé that focuses on your abilities rather than work experience, and it's discussed in detail next.

PARTS OF A RÉSUMÉ

The functional résumé is the best approach when you don't have a lot of pertinent work experience, as it is written to highlight your abilities rather than your experience. (The other, perhaps more common, type of résumé is called the chronological résumé, which lists a person's accomplishments in chronological order, most recent jobs listed first.) This section breaks down and discusses the functional résumé in greater detail.

Here are the essential parts of your résumé, listed from the top down:

- *Heading:* This should include your name, address, and contact information, including phone, e-mail, and website if you have one. This information is typically centered at the top of the page.
- *Objective:* This is a one-sentence statement that tells the employer what kind of position you are seeking. This should be modified to be specific to each potential employer.
- *Education:* Always list your most recent school or program first. Include date of completion (or expected date of graduation), degree or certificate earned, and the institution's name and address. Include workshops, seminars, and related classes here as well.
- *Skills:* Skills include computer literacy, leadership skills, organizational skills, and time-management skills. Be specific in this area when possible.
- *Activities:* Activities can be related to skills. Perhaps an activity listed here helped you develop a skill listed above. This section can be combined with the Skills section, but it's often helpful to break these apart if you have enough substantive things to say in both areas. Examples include sports teams, leadership roles, community service work, clubs and organizations, and so on.

- *Experience:* If you don't have any actual work experience that's relevant, you might consider skipping this section. However, you can list summer, part-time, and volunteer jobs you've held.
- *Interests:* This section is optional, but it's a chance to include special talents and interests. Keep it short, factual, and specific.
- *References:* It's best to say that references are available on request. If you do list actual contacts, list no more than three and make sure you inform your contacts that they might be contacted.

The first three parts above are pretty much standard, but the other entries can be creatively combined or developed to maximize your abilities and experience. These are not set-in-stone sections that every résumé must have. As an example, consider the mock functional résumé on the next page.

If you're still not seeing the big picture here, it's helpful to look at student and part-time résumé examples online to see how others have approached this process. Search for "functional résumé examples" to get a look at some examples.

RÉSUMÉ-WRITING TIPS

Regardless of your situation and why you're writing the résumé, there are some basic tips and techniques you should use:

- Keep it short and simple. This includes using a simple, standard font and format. Using one of the résumé templates included in your word processor software can be a great way to start.
- Use simple language. Keep it to one page.
- Highlight your academic achievements, such as a high GPA (above 3.5) or academic awards. If you have taken classes related to the job you're interviewing for, list those briefly as well.
- Emphasize your extracurricular activities, internships, and the like. These could include clubs, sports, dog walking, babysitting, or volunteer work. Use these activities to show your skills and abilities.
- Use action verbs, such as *led, created, taught, ran,* and *developed.*
- Be specific and give examples.
- Always be honest.
- Include leadership roles and experience.

Robin Jones

620 River Road
Portland, OR, 97035
Phone: 503-503-5030 E-Mail: rwc2004@student.com

Objective

Seeking an entry-level position to further my passion and desire to work with animals in a healthcare setting

Education

High School Diploma, June 2020
Henry James High School, Portland, OR
GPA: 3.94. Top 2% of class

Skills

Computer literacy on PC and Mac; MS Word, Excel, PowerPoint, desktop publishing, web software
Trained in first aid and CPR
Four years of Spanish

Activities

Captain of the Spanish Club, 2020
Outstanding Community Service Award, 2019
Volunteer tutor of Spanish to ESL students, 2018-2019

Experience

2019 co-op volunteer participant, Heartsound Rescue Center, Portland OR
June 2017-June 2019, Part-time volunteer, Heartsound Rescue Center, Portland, OR
May 2016-June 2017, Crew Team Member, Big Burger Stop 'N Eat, Portland, OR

References

Available upon request

A functional résumé is a good template to use when you don't have a lot of work experience.

- Edit and proofread at least twice, and have someone else do the same. Ask a professional (such as your school writing center or your local library services) to proofread it for you also. Don't forget to run spell check.
- Include a cover letter (discussed in the next section).

The Cover Letter

Every résumé you send out should include a cover letter. This can be the most important part of your job search because it's often the first thing that potential employers read. By including the cover letter, you're showing the employers that you took the time to learn about their organization and address them personally. This goes a long way to show that you're interested in the position.

Be sure to call the company or verify on the website the name and title of the person to whom you should address the letter. This letter should be brief. Introduce yourself and begin with a statement that will grab the person's attention. Keep in mind that employers potentially receive hundreds of résumés and cover letters for every open position. You want yours to stand out. Important information to include in the cover letter, from the top, includes:

- The current date
- Your address and contact information
- The person's name, company, and contact information

Then you begin the letter portion of the cover letter, which should mention how you heard about the position, something extra about you that will interest the potential employer, practical skills you can bring to the position, and past experience related to the job. You should apply the facts outlined in your résumé to the job to which you're applying. Each cover letter should be personalized for the position and company to which you're applying. Don't use "To whom it may concern"; instead, take the time to find out to whom you should actually address the letter. Finally, end with a complimentary closing, such as "Sincerely, Henry Smith," and be sure to add your signature. Search for "sample cover letters for internships" or "sample cover letters for high schoolers" to see some good examples.

If you are e-mailing your cover letter instead of printing it out, you'll need to pay particular attention to the subject line of your email. Be sure that it is specific to the position you are applying for. In all cases, it's really important to follow the employer's instructions about how to submit your cover letter and résumé. Generally speaking, sending PDFs rather than editable documents is a better idea. Everyone can read a PDF, but some recipients might not be able to open a document from the particular word-processing program that you used. Most word-processing programs have an option under the Save command that allows you to save your document as a PDF.

> "To avoid burnout, separate your work from your personal life. It's good to be caring and empathetic, but you can't carry those burdens home. Having a good routine for self-care is very important, as it helps relieve emotional stress."—Jia Wang

EFFECTIVELY HANDLING STRESS

As you're forging ahead with your life plans—whether it's college, a full-time job, or even a gap year—you might find that these decisions feel very important and heavy and that the stress is difficult to deal with. This is completely normal. Try these simple techniques to relieve stress:

- Take deep breaths in and out. Try this for thirty seconds. You'll be amazed at how it can help.
- Close your eyes and clear your mind.
- Go scream at the passing subway car. Or lock yourself in a closet and scream. Or scream into a pillow. For some people, this can really help.
- Keep the issue in perspective. Any decision you make now can be changed if it doesn't work out.

Want to know how to avoid stress altogether? It is surprisingly simple. Of course, simple doesn't always mean easy, but these ideas are basic and make sense based on what we know about the human body:

- Get enough sleep.
- Eat healthy.

- Get exercise.
- Go outside.
- Schedule downtime.
- Connect with friends and family.

The bottom line is that you need to take time for self-care. Stress is a part of life, but how you deal with it makes all the difference. This only becomes more important as you enter college or the workforce and maybe have a family. Developing good, consistent habits related to self-care now will serve you all your life.

HELENE PANNWITZ

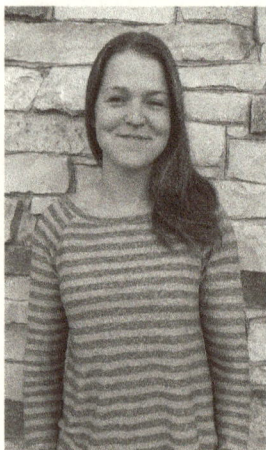

Helene Pannwitz.
Courtesy of Helene Pannwitz

Helene Pannwitz is a veterinary assistant and is working on her associate's degree in veterinary technology. She has worked at the same veterinary hospital as a veterinary assistant since 2006. She also gained experience in high school and during college studies at a general clinic and at a vet hospital as a kennel tech.

Can you explain how you became interested in becoming a vet technician?

I was always interested in veterinary medicine, even as a kid. I just gravitated toward it. It was the only thing I liked.

Can you talk about your current position? What's a typical day in your job?

I currently work in neurology. My day starts with in-house patients and cases in ER that might be transferred to us. Take in appointments in the mornings, helping the doctors with the exams, and typing in the physical exam information and doctor notes. We do a lot of MRIs and surgeries—such as back surgeries. These procedures are more in the afternoon. We deal with cats and dogs mostly—occasionally exotics or zoo, but their specialty techs usually monitor that process.

In neurology, we deal with disk issues, brain abnormalities, tumors and infectious diseases, autoimmune, congenital malformations. We are looking for and ruling out issues with MRIs, blood testing. We do spinal surgeries and craniotomies sometimes, for seizures.

I am very interested in the brain and I worked in the ICW (intensive care ward) previously. I did that for eight or nine years and did overnights. I like the doctors who work in neurology too. It's a mesh between ER and a specialty because neurology sees patients that are emergent. Emergencies that are related to the brain.

Do you think your education prepared you for your job?

My knowledge and technical skills have been honed in the field. There are some times when I don't know the chemistry behind things, because I don't have the full degree yet. Understanding the drugs (such as anesthesia) and understanding the chemistry is a weakness. But otherwise I feel competent. And there is always more to learn.

What's the best part of being a vet technician?

Being able to help animals and their owners. The reward is so much greater than the hard cases, in my opinion. You do get fatigue from seeing hard cases, but the reward is well worth it.

What are some things in this profession that are especially challenging right now?

In neurology specifically, there is no off switch. You work until the work is done. Home life can suffer sometimes because of that.

Overall, the hardest thing is when owners want to do the right thing but they don't have the funds. There are ways to get around that (with Care Credit and payment plans), but sometimes that's the hard reality. I am buffered a little bit from that because most of our patients are referred to us from their general practitioner, so they are usually prepared for the costs by their veterinarian. But it still does happen.

What are some characteristics of a good vet technician?

Good interpersonal skills with coworkers and with patients. Most technicians have to take histories with owners and talk on the phone about patient care. It's not just one-on-one with animals.

A good vet tech also can keep your cool even when the patients aren't doing well. You have to be able to think straight under pressure. There is a lot of skill in restraining an animal without freaking them out. Controlling animals, especially cats, without scaring them is important.

You also have to be somewhat physically fit to pick up and restrain animals. It's a taxing job.

What advice do you have for young people considering this career?

As far as choosing technician over veterinarian, if you like to make decisions and be responsible and can deal with taking cases home with you, veterinarian might be better for you.

The reason I like being a technician is because I get to take part in making an animal better and I get to administer the care, but I am not ultimately responsible for making the final decisions about their care.

Getting your vet tech degree is important and getting your RVT license is important, especially for job mobility.

As far as choosing where to work, such as at a general practice clinic versus a hospital, they both have pros and cons. There is routine at a general practice, such as annual physicals, dental, spays and neuters, dental cleanings, and client education. Hospital work is more interesting and varied, but there are also repeats of similar cases—both are good. A general practice will mean more structured hours probably. You'll see more serious conditions at a hospital.

How can a young person prepare for a career as a vet technician while in high school?

Volunteer at a veterinary hospital or clinic or humane society or other shelters and rescues while in school to get experience working with animals.

What are your future plans?

I love it and will stick with it. It's very rewarding. There aren't very many days when I question what I do. There are also emerging specialties within the technician field, so there is growth capability that way.

Any last thoughts?

Many people are afraid of the career path because of euthanasia. But it's not always the wrong or bad choice. The upside is that it's a gift for patients that are suffering. It's a loving choice. So it can have an upside. Also, doctors have a choice and can refuse to put the animal down just because the owners are moving and they don't want it anymore. We have some control over that.

Interviewing Skills

The best way to avoid nerves and keep calm when you're interviewing is to be prepared. It's okay to feel scared, but keep it in perspective. It's likely that you'll receive many more rejections than acceptances in your professional life, as we all do. However, you only need one *yes* to start out. Think of the interviewing process as a learning experience. With the right attitude, you will learn from each one and get better with each subsequent interview. That should be your overarching goal. Consider these tips and tricks when interviewing, whether it be for a job, internship, college admission, or something else entirely:

- Practice interviewing with a friend or relative. Practicing will help calm your nerves and make you feel more prepared. Ask for specific feedback from your friends. Do you need to speak more loudly? Are you making enough eye contact? Are you actively listening when the other person is speaking?
- Learn as much as you can about the company, school, or organization, and be sure to understand the position for which you're applying. This will show the interviewer that you are motivated and interested in the organization.
- Speak up during the interview. Convey to the interviewer important points about yourself. Don't be afraid to ask questions. Try to remember the interviewers' names and call them by name.
- Arrive early and dress professionally and appropriately. (You can read more about proper dress in a following section.)
- Take some time to prepare answers to commonly asked questions. Be ready to describe your career or educational goals to the interviewer.[1]

Common questions you may be asked during a job interview include:

- Tell me about yourself.
- What are your greatest strengths?
- What are your weaknesses?
- Tell me something about yourself that's not on your résumé.
- What are your career goals?
- How do you handle failure? Are you willing to fail?

- How do you handle stress and pressure?
- What are you passionate about?
- Why do you want to work for us?

Common questions you may be asked during a college admissions interview include these:

- Tell me about yourself.
- Why are you interested in going to college?
- Why do you want to major in this subject?
- What are your academic strengths?
- What are your academic weaknesses? How have you addressed them?
- What will you contribute to this college/school/university?
- Where do you see yourself in ten years?
- How do you handle failure? Are you willing to fail?
- How do you handle stress and pressure?
- Whom do you most admire?
- What is your favorite book?
- What do you do for fun?
- Why are you interested in this college/school/university?

Jot down notes about your answers to these questions, but don't try to memorize the answers. You don't want to come off as too rehearsed during the interview. Remember to be as specific and detailed as possible when answering these questions. Your goal is to set yourself apart in some way from the other interviewees. Always accentuate the positive, even when you're asked about something you did not like, or about failure or stress. Most importantly, though, be yourself.

Active listening is the process of fully concentrating on what is being said, understanding it, and providing nonverbal cues and responses to the person talking.[2] It's the opposite of being distracted and thinking about something else when someone is talking. Active listening takes practice. You might find that your mind wanders and you need to bring your attention back to the person talking (and this could happen multiple times during one conversation). Practice this technique in regular conversations with friends and relatives. In addition to giving a better interview, it can cut down on nerves and make you more popular with friends and family, as everyone wants to feel that they are really being heard. For more on active listening, check out www .mindtools.com/CommSkll/ActiveListening.htm.

You should also be ready to ask questions of your interviewer. In a practical sense, there should be some questions you have that you can't find the answer to on the website or in the literature. Also, asking questions shows that you are interested and have done your homework. Avoid asking questions about salary, scholarships, or special benefits at this stage, and don't ask about anything negative that you've heard about the company or school. Keep the questions positive and related to the position to which you're applying. Some example questions to potential employers include:

- What is a typical career path for a person in this position?
- How would you describe the ideal candidate for this position?
- How is the department organized?
- What kind of responsibilities come with this job? (Don't ask this if it has already been addressed in the job description or discussion.)
- What can I do as a follow-up?
- When do you expect to reach a decision?

See "Making the Most of Campus Visits" in chapter 3 for some good examples of questions to ask the college admissions office. The important thing is to write your own questions related to information you really want to know, and be sure your question isn't already answered on the website, in the job description, or in the literature. This will show genuine interest.

Dressing Appropriately

It's important to determine what is actually appropriate in the setting of the interview. What is appropriate in a corporate setting might be different from what you'd expect at a small liberal arts college or at a large hospital setting. For example, most college admissions offices suggest business casual attire, but

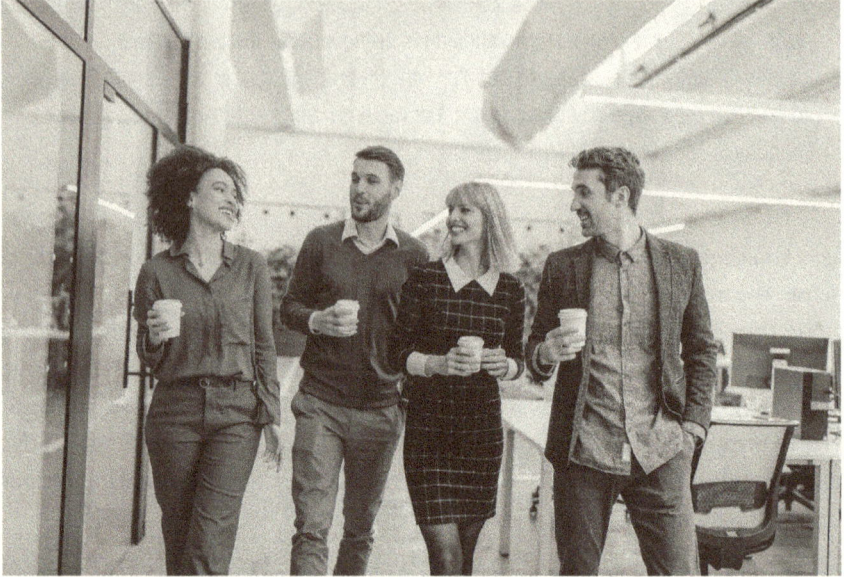

Even something like "business casual" can be interpreted in many ways, so do some research to find out what exactly is expected of you. ©*bernardbodo/iStock/Getty Images*

depending on the job interview, you may want to step it up from there. Again, it's important to do your homework and be prepared. In addition to reading up on organization's guidelines, it never hurts to take a look around the website if you can to see what other people are wearing to work or to interviews. Regardless of the setting, make sure your clothes are not wrinkled, untidy, or stained. Avoid flashy clothing of any kind.

Follow-Up Communication

Be sure to follow up, whether via e-mail or regular mail, with a thank-you note to the interviewer. This is true whether you're interviewing for a job or internship or interviewing with a college. A handwritten thank-you note, posted in the mail, is best. In addition to showing consideration, it will trigger the interviewer's memory about you and it shows that you have genuine interest in the position, company, or school. Be sure to follow the business letter format and highlight the key points of your interview and experience at the company or school. And be prompt with your thank-you note! Put it in the mail the day after your interview or send it by email the same day.

What Employers Expect

Regardless of the job, profession, or field, there are universal characteristics that all employers—and schools, for that matter—look for in candidates. At this early stage in your professional life, you have an opportunity to recognize which of these foundational characteristics are your strengths (and therefore highlight them in an interview) and which are weaknesses (and therefore continue to work on them and build them up). Consider these characteristics:

- Positive attitude
- Dependability
- Desire to continue to learn
- Initiative
- Effective communication
- Cooperation
- Organization

This is not an exhaustive list, and other desirable characteristics include things like sensitivity to others, honesty, good judgment, loyalty, responsibility, and punctuality. Specific to healthcare/veterinary medicine, you can add having empathy, attention to detail, flexibility, having a caring nature, and being organized to that list. Consider these important characteristics when you answer the common questions that employers ask. It pays to work these traits into the answers—of course, being honest and realistic about your traits.

Beware the social media trap! Prospective employers and colleges will check your social media profiles, so make sure there is nothing too personal, explicit, or inappropriate out there. When you communicate to the world on social media, don't use profanity—and be sure to use proper grammar. Think about the version of yourself you are portraying online. Is it favorable or at least neutral to potential employers? Rest assured: they will look.

Personal contacts can make the difference! Don't be afraid to contact people you know. Personal connections can be a great way to find jobs and internship opportunities. Your high school teachers, your coaches and mentors, and your friends' parents are all examples of people who very well may know about jobs or internships that would suit you. Start asking several months before you hope to start a job or internship, because it will take some time to do research and arrange interviews. You can also use social media in your search. LinkedIn (www.linkedin.com), for example, includes lots of searchable information on local companies. Follow and interact with people on social media to get their attention. Just remember to act professionally and communicate with proper grammar, just as you would in person.

Summary

Well, you made it to the end of this book! Hopefully, you have learned enough about the vet technician field to start along your journey or to continue along your path. If you've reached the end and you feel like paraveterinary medicine is right for you, that's great news. If you've figured out that this isn't the right field for you, that's good information to learn, too. For many of us, figuring out what we *don't* want to do and what we *don't* like is an important step in finding the right career.

There is a lot of good news about the paraveterinary medicine field, and it's a smart career choice for anyone with a passion to help animals. It's fulfilling, flexible, and certainly not monotonous. Job demand is high and will continue to grow in the foreseeable future.

"This profession is not at all what I expected. To me, it's better! You don't just hold the animals while the doctors examine them, which is what I thought originally. You do much more hands-on work with the animals—including giving shots, taking blood, cleaning teeth, giving vaccines, acting as a receptionist, talking to owners, and restraining and comforting animals. It's really hands-on—and rewarding!"—Krista King

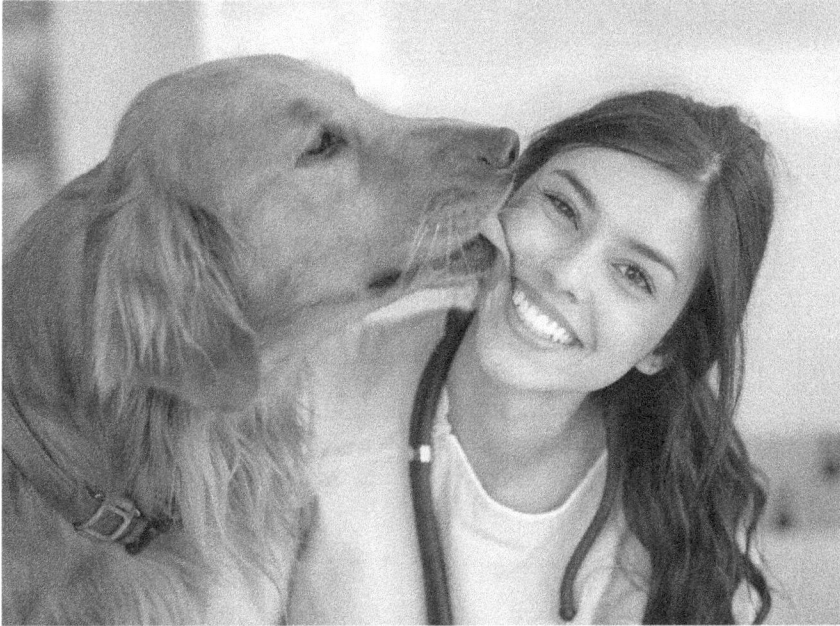

With a little hard work and perseverance, you'll be on your way to career success, no matter how you measure it! ©*andresr/E+/Getty Images*

Whether you decide to attend a four-year university, get an associate's degree, take a gap year, or do something else entirely, having a plan and an idea about your future can help guide your decisions. After reading this book, you should be well on your way to having a plan for your future. Good luck to you as you move ahead!

Notes

Introduction

1. Barry Franklin, "Veterinary Technician vs. Veterinary Technologist," VetTech Colleges, https://www.vettechcolleges.com/blog/veterinary-technician-vs-technologist.

2. Bureau of Labor Statistics, Occupational Outlook Handbook, https://www.bls.gov/ooh/healthcare/veterinary-technologists-and-technicians.htm.

3. Bureau of Labor Statistics, US Department of Labor, "Veterinary Technologists and Technicians," https://www.bls.gov/ooh/healthcare/veterinary-technologists-and-technicians.htm.

4. Ibid.

Chapter 1: Why Choose a Career as a Veterinary Technician or Assistant?

1. The Balance Careers, "What Does a Veterinary Assistant Do?" https://www.thebalancecareers.com/what-is-a-veterinary-assistant-526079.

2. Adapted from Bureau of Labor Statistics, US Department of Labor, "Veterinary Assistants and Laboratory Animal Caretakers: Summary," https://www.bls.gov/ooh/healthcare/veterinary-assistants-and-laboratory-animal-caretakers.htm#tab-1.

3. Truity, "Veterinary Technologist or Technician," https://www.truity.com/career-profile/veterinary-technologist-or-technician.

4. Bureau of Labor Statistics, US Department of Labor, "Veterinary Technologists and Technicians," https://www.bls.gov/ooh/healthcare/veterinary-technologists-and-technicians.htm.

5. Ibid.

6. Adapted from Bureau of Labor Statistics, US Department of Labor, "Veterinary Technologists and Technicians: Work Environment," https://www.bls.gov/ooh/healthcare/veterinary-technologists-and-technicians.htm#tab-3.

7. VetTech Colleges, "Veterinary Technician vs. Veterinary Technologist," https://www.vettechcolleges.com/blog/veterinary-technician-vs-technologist.

8. American Veterinary Medical Association, "AVMA Policy on Veterinary Technology," https://www.avma.org/KB/Policies/Pages/AVMA-Policy-on-Veterinary -Technology.aspx.

9. CindyRVT, "Difference between Vet Technician and Vet Technologist?" Comments on Indeed.com Forums, https://www.indeed.com/forum/job/veterinary -technician/Difference-between-vet-technician-vet-technologist/t384922.

10. Truity, "Veterinary Technologist or Technician," https://www.truity.com /career-profile/veterinary-technologist-or-technician.

11. The Balance Careers, "What Does a Veterinary Technician Do?" https ://www.thebalancecareers.com/what-is-a-veterinary-technician-526080.

12. Academy of Veterinary Behavior Technicians, "Become a Specialist," https ://avbt.net/membership.

13. National Academy of Veterinary Technicians in America, "Specialties," https://www.navta.net/page/specialties.

14. Veterinary Emergency and Critical Care Society, "Certification Levels," http://veccs.org/facility-certification/certification-levels.

15. American Association of Equine Veterinary Technicians and Assistants, "Specialties," https://www.aaevt.org/online-certificate-program/.

16. Academy of Internal Medicine for Veterinary Technicians, "Core Applications Instructions," https://www.aimvt.com/core-requirements.html.

17. National Association of Veterinary Technicians in America, "Specialties."

18. Academy of Veterinary Surgical Technicians, "Requirements to Apply," http://www.avst-vts.org/requirements.html.

19. Veterinary Technician Schools, "Veterinary Technician Anesthetist," http ://www.veterinarytechnicianinfo.com/veterinary-technician-anesthetist.

20. Academy of Veterinary Dental Technicians, "Credentialing Guidelines," https://www.avdt.us/credentialing-guidelines.

21. American Academy of Veterinary Nutrition, "Student Resources," https ://acvn.org/student-resources.

22. Association of Zoo Veterinary Technicians, "How Do I Become a Zoo Veterinary Technician?" https://www.azvt.org/page-18118.

Chapter 2: Forming a Career Plan

1. Truity, "Veterinary Technologist or Technician," https://www.truity.com /career-profile/veterinary-technologist-or-technician.

2. American Veterinary Medical Association, "Who We Are," https://www.avma.org/About/WhoWeAre/Pages/default.aspx.

3. American Veterinary Medical Association, "Programs accredited by the AVMA Committee on Veterinary Technician Education and Activities (CVTEA)," https://www.avma.org/ProfessionalDevelopment/Education/Accreditation/Programs/Pages/vettech-programs.aspx.

4. Ibid.

5. American Association of Veterinary State Boards, "Veterinary Technician National Exam (VTNE)," https://www.aavsb.org/vtne-overview.

6. Online Schools Center, "What Is the Difference between Being a Veterinary Assistant, Technician, or Technologist?" https://www.onlineschoolscenter.com/difference-veterinary-assistant-technician-technologist.

7. LinkedIn.com, "New Survey Reveals 85% of All Jobs are Filled Via Networking," www.linkedin.com/pulse/new-survey-reveals-85-all-jobs-filled-via-networking-lou-adler.

8. NewGradPhysicalTherapy.com, "Leverage Your Volunteering Experience," https://newgradphysicaltherapy.com/volunteer-experience-physical-therapy-school.

Chapter 3: Pursuing the Education Path

1. Peter Van Buskirk, "Finding a Good College Fit," *U.S. News & World Report*, June 13, 2011, https://www.usnews.com/education/blogs/the-college-admissions-insider/2011/06/13/finding-a-good-college-fit.

2. National Center for Education Statistics, "Fast Facts: Graduation Rates," https://nces.ed.gov/fastfacts/display.asp?id=40.

3. US Department of Education, "Focusing Higher Education on Student Success," July 27, 2015, https://www.ed.gov/news/press-releases/factsheet-focusing-higher-education-student-success.

4. CindyRVT, "Difference between Vet Technician and Vet Technologist?" Comments on Indeed.com Forums, https://www.indeed.com/forum/job/veterinary-technician/Difference-between-vet-technician-vet-technologist/t384922.

5. National Center for Education Statistics, "Fast Facts: Tuition Costs of Colleges and Universities," https://nces.ed.gov/programs/digest/d18/tables/dt18_330.20.asp.

6. College Board, "Understanding College Costs," https://bigfuture.collegeboard.org/pay-for-college/college-costs/understanding-college-costs.

7. Gap Year Association, "Research Statement," https://gapyearassociation.org/research.php.

8. Federal Student Aid, "7 Things You Need before You Fill Out the 2020–21 FAFSA Form," *HomeRoom: The Official Blog of the US Department of Education*, September 10, 2019, https://blog.ed.gov/2019/09/7-things-need-fill-2020-21-fafsa-form.

Chapter 4: Writing Your Résumé and Interviewing

1. Justin Ross Muchnick, *Teens' Guide to College & Career Planning*, 12th ed. (Lawrenceville, NJ: Peterson's, 2015), 179–80.

2. Mind Tools, "Active Listening: Hear What People Are Really Saying," https://www.mindtools.com/CommSkll/ActiveListening.htm.

Glossary

accreditation: The act of officially recognizing an organizational body, person, or educational facility as having a particular status or being qualified to perform a particular activity. For example, schools and colleges are accredited. *See also* **certification**.

ACT: One of the standardized college entrance tests that anyone wanting to enter undergraduate studies in the United States should take. It measures knowledge and skills in mathematics, English, reading, and science reasoning as they apply to college readiness. There are four multiple-choice sections and an optional writing test. The total score of the ACT is 36. *See also* **SAT**.

American Veterinary Medical Association (AVMA): A not-for-profit association representing more than ninety-three thousand veterinarians working in private and corporate practice, government, industry, academia, and uniformed services. The AVMA acts as a collective voice for its membership and for the profession.

American Veterinary Technician National Examination (VTNE): Most states require veterinary technicians to pass this test, which is given three times a year. (Note that each state regulates veterinary technologists and technicians differently.) The computer-based exam is given at testing centers throughout the United States and Canada.

anatomy: The area of science concerned with the bodily structure and organization of humans, animals, and other living things.

anesthesia: Medicine that is given to patients so that surgery and other medical processes can be performed without causing them any pain; and in many situations, patients are not awake or conscious during the procedure. There are many of types of anesthesia.

associate's degree: A degree awarded by a community or junior college that typically requires two years of study. Vet technicians typically earn an associate's degree.

bachelor's degree: An undergraduate degree awarded by a college or university that is typically a four-year course of study when pursued full-time, but this can vary by the degree earned and by the university awarding the degree. Vet technologists typically earn a bachelor's degree.

cardiovascular system: The system of the body making up the heart and blood, including veins and arteries. Applicable diseases include stroke, heart attack, and high blood pressure.

certification: The action or process of confirming that an individual has acquired certain skills or knowledge, usually provided by some third-party review, assessment, or educational body. Individuals, not organizations, are certified. *See also* **accreditation**.

diagnosis: When a healthcare professional determines the nature of an illness or problem after examining a patient.

doctorate degree: The highest level of degree awarded by colleges and universities. This degree qualifies the holder to teach at the university level and requires (usually published) research in the field. Earning a doctoral degree typically requires an additional three to five years of study after earning a bachelor's degree. Anyone with a doctorate degree—not just medical doctors—can be addressed as "Doctor."

euthanize: The act of putting a living being to death humanely, without pain.

fear-free movement: A movement that focuses on providing pets with calming environments to help alleviate fear, anxiety, and stress, particularly when visiting the veterinarian's office. Started in 2016 by Dr. Marty Becker, the organization Fear Free provides education and certifications in fear-free practices.

gap year: A gap year is a year between high school and college (or sometimes between college and postgraduate studies) during which the student is not in school but is instead typically involved in other pursuits, typically a volunteer program such as the Peace Corps or AmeriCorps, travel, or work and teaching.

grants: Money to pay for postsecondary education that is typically awarded to students who have financial need, but can also be used in the areas of athletics, academics, demographics, veteran support, and special talents. Grants do not have to be paid back.

license: An official document, card, certificate, or the like that gives you permission to have, use, or do something, such as to practice as a vet technician. Typically, one gets certified and then applies for a license.

master's degree: A postgraduate degree awarded by colleges and universities that requires at least one additional year of study after obtaining a bachelor's degree. The degree holder shows mastery of a specific field.

paraveterinary worker: An umbrella term that refers to vet technicians, vet technologists, and vet assistants. These are professionals who assist veterinary physicians in the performance of their duties and otherwise carry out animal health procedures as part of a veterinary care system.

pathology: The science that identifies and manages diseases.

personal statement: A written description of your accomplishments, outlook, interests, goals, and personality that is an important part of your college application. The personal statement should set you apart from other applicants. The required length depends on the institution, but they generally range from one to two pages, or 500–1,000 words.

postsecondary degree: An educational degree above and beyond a high school education. This is a general description that includes trade certificates and certifications; associate's, bachelor's, and master's degrees; and beyond.

rehabilitation: The process of returning a patient to a healthier state, better health, or a more functional life after an illness or accident.

SAT: One of the standardized tests in the United States that anyone applying to undergraduate studies should take. It measures verbal and mathematical reasoning abilities as they relate to predicting successful performance in college. It is intended to complement a student's GPA and school record in assessing readiness for college. The total score of the SAT is 1600. *See also* **ACT**.

scholarships: Merit-based aid used to pay for postsecondary education that does not have to be paid back. Scholarships are typically awarded based on academic excellence or some other special talent, such as music or art.

veterinary assistant: An individual who performs duties such as feeding and exercising animals, bathing animals and cleaning their cages, comforting and restraining animals during procedures, and otherwise assisting veterinarians and vet technicians. Working as a vet assistant requires a high school diploma only.

veterinary technician: A graduate from a two-year AVMA-accredited program from a community college, college, or university. Vet technicians generally work in private clinical practices or hospitals under the guidance of a licensed veterinarian.

veterinary technologist: A graduate from a four-year AVMA-accredited bachelor's degree program. Many vet technologists work in more advanced, research-related jobs, usually under the guidance of a scientist and sometimes a veterinarian; they primarily work in laboratory settings.

Resources

Are you looking for more information about the paraveterinary medicine field or even about a branch within healthcare in general? Do you want to know more about the college application process or need some help finding the right educational fit for you? Do you want a quick way to search for a good college or school? Try these resources as a starting point on your journey toward finding a great career!

Books

Bassert, Joanna M. *McCurnin's Clinical Textbook for Veterinary Technicians*, 9th ed. St. Louis, MO: Elsevier Books, 2018.

Field, Shelly. *Career Opportunities in Health Care*, 3rd ed. New York: Checkmark Books, 2007.

Fiske, Edward. *Fiske Guide to Colleges*. Naperville, IL: Sourcebooks, 2018.

Muchnick, Justin Ross. *Teens' Guide to College & Career Planning*, 12th ed. Lawrenceville, NJ: Peterson's, 2015.

Princeton Review. *The Best 382 Colleges, 2018 Edition: Everything You Need to Make the Right College Choice*. New York: Princeton Review, 2018.

Websites

American Gap Year Association
www.gapyearassociation.org
The American Gap Year Association's mission is "making transformative gap years an accessible option for all high school graduates." A gap year is a year taken between high school and college to travel, teach, work, volunteer, generally mature, and otherwise experience the world. The website has lots of advice and resources for anyone considering taking a gap year.

American Veterinary Medical Association (AVMA)
www.avma.org
Includes information about professional development, meetings, and events; links to AVMA journals; and an updated list of vet tech programs that have been accredited by the CVTEA, the accrediting arm of the AVMA. The site provides links to each state so you can see the accredited programs in your area.

The Balance
www.thebalance.com
This site is all about managing money and finances, but also has a large section called Your Career, which provides advice for writing résumés and cover letters, interviewing, and more. Search the site for teens and you can find teen-specific advice and tips.

The College Entrance Examination Board
www.collegeboard.org
The College Entrance Examination Board tracks and summarizes financial data from colleges and universities all over the United States. This great, well-organized site can be your one-stop shop for all things college research. It contains lots of advice and information about taking and doing well on the SAT and ACT tests, many articles on college planning, a robust college searching feature, a scholarship searching feature, and a major and career search area. You can type your career of interest (for example, veterinary technician) into the search box and get back a full page that describes the career; gives advice on how to prepare, where to get experience, and how to pay for it; what characteristics you should have to excel in this career; lists of helpful classes to take while in high school; and lots of links for more information.

College Grad Career Profiles
www.collegegrad.com/careers
Although this site is primarily geared toward college graduates, the career profiles area, indicated above, has a list of links to nearly every career you could ever think of. A single click takes you to a very helpful section that describes the job in detail, explains the educational requirements, includes links to good colleges that offer this career and to actual open jobs and internships, describes the licensing requirements (if any), lists salaries, and much more.

Explore Health Careers Website

www.explorehealthcareers.org

As the title suggests, this site enables you to explore careers in the health fields. You can seek answers to questions such as whether a career in health is right for you, find the right fit and focus your search within the many fields, actually find the job or internship you're looking for, learn more about paying for college, and more.

Khan Academy

www.khanacademy.org

The Khan Academy website is an impressive collection of articles, courses, and videos about many educational topics in math, science, and the humanities. You can search any topic or subject (by subject matter and grade), and read lessons, take courses, and watch videos to learn all about it. The site includes test prep information for the SAT, ACT, AP, GMAT, and other standardized tests. There is also a College Admissions tab with lots of good articles and information, provided in the approachable Khan style.

Live Career Website

www.livecareer.com

This site has an impressive number of resources directed toward teens for writing résumés and cover letters, as well as interviewing.

Mapping Your Future

www.mappingyourfuture.org

This site helps young people figure out what they want to do and maps out how to reach career goals. Includes helpful tips on résumé writing, job hunting, job interviewing, and more.

Monster.com

www.monster.com

Monster.com is perhaps the most well-known and certainly one of the largest employment websites in the United States. You fill in a couple of search boxes and away you go. You can sort by job title, of course, as well as by company name, location, salary range, experience range, and much more. The site also includes information about career fairs, advice on résumés and interviewing, and more.

National Association of Veterinary Technicians in America (NAVTA)
www.navta.net
NAVTA's mission is to advance veterinary nursing and veterinary technology. Its website includes lots of information about the veterinary specialties as well as information about vet technician and vet assistant programs and requirements. You can also connect to state-specific information and resources from this site and find resources for physical and mental health issues related to the occupation.

Occupational Outlook Handbook
www.bls.gov
The US Bureau of Labor Statistics produces this website, which offers lots of relevant and updated information about various careers, including average salaries, how to work in the industry, job market outlook, typical work environments, and what workers do on the job. See www.bls.gov/emp for a full list of employment projections.

Peterson's College Prep
www.petersons.com
In addition to lots of information about preparing for the ACT and SAT and easily searchable information about scholarships nationwide, the Peterson's site includes a comprehensive search feature for universities and schools based on location, major, name, and more.

Study.com
www.study.com
Similar to Khan Academy, Study.com allows you to search any topic or subject and read lessons, take courses, and watch videos to learn all about it. The site includes a good collection of information about basic science and biology needed to excel in vet tech school.

TeenLife
www.teenlife.com
This site calls itself "the leading source for college preparation," and it includes lots of information about summer programs, gap year programs, community service, and more. Promoting the belief that spending time out "in the world"

outside of the classroom can help students develop important life skills, this site contains lots of links to volunteer and summer programs.

U.S. News & World Report *College Rankings*
www.usnews.com/best-colleges
U.S. News & World Report provides almost fifty different types of numerical rankings and lists of colleges throughout the United States to help students with their college search. You can search colleges by best reviewed, best value for the money, best liberal arts schools, best schools for B students, and more.

About the Author

Kezia Endsley is an editor and author from Indianapolis, Indiana. In addition to editing technical publications and writing books for teens, she enjoys running and triathlons, traveling, reading, and spending time with her family and seven pets.

www.ingramcontent.com/pod-product-compliance
Lightning Source LLC
Chambersburg PA
CBHW021822270326
41932CB00007B/296